KU-686-391

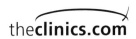
theclinics.com

UROLOGIC CLINICS

OF NORTH AMERICA

Office Management and
Procedures

GUEST EDITOR
William F. Gee, MD

CONSULTING EDITOR
Martin I. Resnick, MD

August 2005 • Volume 32 • Number 3

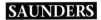
SAUNDERS

An Imprint of Elsevier, Inc.
PHILADELPHIA   LONDON   TORONTO   MONTREAL   SYDNEY   TOKYO

W.B. SAUNDERS COMPANY
A Division of Elsevier Inc.

1600 John F. Kennedy Boulevard • Suite 1800 • Philadelphia, Pennsylvania 19103-2899

http://www.theclinics.com

THE UROLOGIC CLINICS OF NORTH AMERICA
August 2005
Editor: Catherine Bewick

Volume 32, Number 3
ISSN 0094-0143
ISBN 1-4160-2802-1

Copyright © 2005 Elsevier Inc. All rights reserved. No part of this publication may be reproduced or transmitted in any form or by any means, electronic or mechanical, including photocopy, recording, or any information retrieval system, without written permission from the Publisher.

Single photocopies of single articles may be made for personal use as allowed by national copyright laws. Permission of the Publisher and payment of a fee is required for all other photocopying, including multiple or systematic copying, copying for advertising or promotional purposes, resale, and all forms of document delivery. Special rates are available for educational institutions that wish to make photocopies for non-profit educational classroom use. Permissions may be sought directly from Elsevier's Rights Department in Philadelphia, PA, USA; phone: (+1) 215 239 3804, fax: (+1) 215 239 3805, e-mail: healthpermissions@elsevier.com. Requests may also be completed online via the Elsevier homepage (http://www.elsevier.com/locate/permissions). In the USA, users may clear permissions and make payments through the Copyright Clearance Center, Inc., 222 Rosewood Drive, Danvers, MA 01923, USA; phone: (978) 750-8400, fax: (978) 750-4744, and in the UK through the copyright Licensing Agency Rapid Clearance Service (CLARCS), 90 Tottenham Court Road, London W1P 0LP, UK; phone: (+44) 171 436 5931; fax: (+44) 171 436 3986. Other countries may have a local reprographic rights agency for payments.

Reprints. For copies of 100 or more, of articles in this publication, please contact the Commercial Reprints Department, Elsevier Inc., 360 Park Avenue South, New York, New York 10010-1710. Tel.: (212) 633-3813, Fax: (212) 462-1935, e-mail: reprints@elsevier.com.

The ideas and opinions expressed in *The Urologic Clinics of North America* do not necessarily reflect those of the Publisher. The Publisher does not assume any responsibility for any injury and/or damage to persons or property arising out of or related to any use of the material contained in this periodical. The reader is advised to check the appropriate medical literature and the product information currently provided by the manufacturer of each drug to be administered to verify the dosage, the method and duration of administration, or contraindications. It is the responsibility of the treating physician or other health care professional, relying on independent experience and knowledge of the patient, to determine drug dosages and the best treatment for the patient. Mention of any product in this issue should not be construed as endorsement by the contributors, editors, or the Publisher of the product or manufacturers' claims.

The Urologic Clinics of North America (ISSN 0094-0143) is published quarterly by W.B. Saunders Company. Corporate and editorial offices: Elsevier, Inc., 1600 John F. Kennedy Blvd., Suite 1800, Philadelphia, PA 19103-2899. Accounting and circulation offices: 6277 Sea Harbor Drive, Orlando, FL 32887-4800. Periodicals postage paid at Orlando, FL 32862, and additional mailing offices. Subscription prices are $195.00 per year (US individuals), $307.00 per year (US institutions), $225.00 per year (Canadian individuals), $371.00 per year (Canadian institutions), $260.00 per year (foreign individuals), and $371.00 per year (foreign institutions). Foreign air speed delivery is included in all *Clinics* subscription prices. All prices are subject to change without notice. POSTMASTER: Send address changes to *The Urologic Clinics of North America*, W.B. Saunders Company, Periodicals Fulfillment, Orlando, FL 32887-4800. **Customer Service: 1-800-654-2452 (US). From outside the US, call 1-407-345-4000.**

The Urologic Clinics of North America is covered in *Index Medicus, Excerpta Medica, Current Contents/ Clinical Medicine, Science Citation Index,* and *ISI/BIOMED*.

Printed in the United States of America.

CONSULTING EDITOR

MARTIN I. RESNICK, MD, Lester Persky Professor and Chairman, Department of Urology, Case Western Reserve University, School of Medicine/University Hospitals, Cleveland, Ohio

GUEST EDITOR

WILLIAM F. GEE, MD, Managing Partner, Commonwealth Urology; and Associate Clinical Professor of Urology (Surgery), University of Kentucky, Lexington, Kentucky

CONTRIBUTORS

JOSEPH W. AKORNOR, MD, Resident Physician, Department of Urology, Mayo Clinic, Rochester, Minnesota

DAVID M. ANDREW, JD, Member, Hemmer Pangburn DeFrank PLLC, Ft. Mitchell, Kentucky

FATIH ATUG, MD, Fellow, Department of Urology, Tulane University Health Sciences Center, New Orleans, Louisiana

NEIL BAUM, MD, Associate Clinical Professor of Urology, Tulane University School of Medicine, New Orleans, Louisiana

JOEL M. BLAU, CFP^{TM}, President, MEDIQUS Asset Advisors, Inc., Chicago, Illinois

ERIK P. CASTLE, MD, Assistant Professor, Department of Urology, Tulane University Health Sciences Center, New Orleans, Louisiana

EMILY E. COLE, MD, Department of Urologic Surgery, Vanderbilt University Medical Center, Nashville, Tennessee

ROGER R. DMOCHOWSKI, MD, FACS, Department of Urologic Surgery, Vanderbilt University Medical Center, Nashville, Tennessee

VIKRAM DOGRA, MD, Associate Chair for Education and Research; Director, Division of Ultrasound; and Professor of Diagnostic Radiology, Department of Imaging Sciences, University of Rochester Medical Center, Rochester, New York

NICK A. FABRIZIO, PhD, Practice Administrator and Assistant Professor, Department of Family Medicine, Upstate Medical University, SUNY at Syracuse; and Independent Consultant, Medical Group Management Association, Health Care Consulting Group, Syracuse, New York

KENNETH T. HERTZ, Independent Consultant, Medical Group Management Association, Health Care Consulting Group, Alexandria, Louisiana

PAULITA A. KEITH, CPA, Healthcare Practice Consultants, LLC, Louisville, Kentucky

SARAH E. McACHRAN, MD, Resident, Department of Urology, Case Western Reserve University, School of Medicine, Cleveland, Ohio

AJAY NEHRA, MD, FACS, Professor of Urology, Department of Urology, Mayo Clinic College of Medicine, Rochester, Minnesota

MARTIN I. RESNICK, MD, Lester Persky Professor and Chairman, Department of Urology, Case Western Reserve University, School of Medicine/University Hospitals, Cleveland, Ohio

RICK RUTHERFORD, CMPE, American Urological Association, Linthicum, Maryland

JOSEPH W. SEGURA, MD, Carl Rosen Professor of Urology, Department of Urology, Mayo Clinic College of Medicine, Rochester, Minnesota

CINDY SPEARS, Healthcare Consultant, Dean, Dorton & Ford, PSC, Lexington, Kentucky

STEPHANIE N. STINCHCOMB, CPC, CCS-P, Coding and Reimbursement Coordinator, Practice Management Department, American Urological Association, Linthicum, Maryland

RAJU THOMAS, MD, FACS, MHA, Professor and Chairman, Department of Urology, Tulane University Health Sciences Center, New Orleans, Louisiana

CONTRIBUTORS

CONTENTS

Most employers eventually face personnel and employment issues. For a medical practice without the resources of a major company, personnel and employment questions present an array of concerns and potential pitfalls. This article presents an overview of personnel and employment issues frequently encountered by medical practices, including the Family and Medical Leave Act, the Americans with Disability Act, the Civil Rights Act of 1964, the Age Discrimination in Employment Act, and handling personnel issues. The article's intent is to provide an understanding of some basic personnel and employment law issues and ways to manage the issues.

A business accountant should be a trusted business advisor and not-so-silent partner. Accountants can assist in making the ordinary everyday decisions in a practice, such as type of business entity under which to operate; type of compensation model a practice should use; type of funding strategy that should be used for capital improvements (eg, leasing versus buying); depreciation methods that should be used; tax strategies for maximizing deductions; retirement plan strategies; practice growth strategies; and many other practice decisions.

During most of the twentieth century, physicians were in charge of their own reimbursements for services. Before the 1980s, there were few mandates or regulations regarding the services they provided, no bundling issues, no modifiers, and no written referrals. Physicians and their staff focused on healing patients, not on a business plan. The end of the century brought challenges and a different environment for health care providers. One of these is the responsibility of physicians to negotiate insurance contracts. This article outlines the ways to negotiate an insurance contract successfully.

Medical Records Management—Steps Toward a Paperless Environment 275
Rick Rutherford

Urologists will be driven slowly but surely toward using electronic health records, even in small practices. This article shows a picture of the current landscape, highlights the paths to adoption, and reassures readers that despite the pain associated with change, using electronic processes to manage health care information can provide cost reductions, improvement in quality, and an increased percentage of time in direct patient care. The environment is changing rapidly and urologists must stay aware and be prepared to make good strategic decisions based on rapidly changing information. There is risk but also great reward if they are done right.

Coding and Reimbursement: The Lifeline of the Urologist's Office 285
Stephanie N. Stinchcomb

Coding rules and regulations change constantly, and this issue of *Urologic Clinics of North America* is not intended to be a coding and reimbursement course. Hopefully, all readers of this issue periodically send their staff (physicians and coders) to courses to learn the latest wrinkles in coding. Accurate coding depends on the information sources that the coding staff has available. A valuable and comprehensive compilation of information resources is included at the end of this article.

Strategic Planning and Budgeting 291
Nick A. Fabrizio and Kenneth T. Hertz

Medical groups must take the time to inventory their current short-term strategy, measure their success, and make course corrections along the way in a proactive methodological process. At the same time, it is important to develop a long-term strategy for market share and profitability. The strategic planning process is a way for groups to satisfy current and future needs while solidifying the group's mission, vision, and harmony. Budgeting is an integral part of the medical practice's long and short term planning process. Budget development requires a deep and thorough understanding of a practice's infrastructure, its operations and processes. In addition to the creation of financial goals, the budget process insures that the management team, and physician leadership continue to be well informed regarding the practice's health.

Marketing Your Urologic Practice—Ethically, Effectively, and Economically 299
Neil Baum

Marketing is an essential ingredient for every successful urologic practice. There are four components of a marketing program: maintaining patients who already are in the practice; attracting new patients; motivating staff to take care of the patients; and providing excellent communication with referring physicians and other health care professionals. All of these marketing components can be achieved with existing staff and with minimal expense. By using marketing techniques, urologists can sculpt the exact kind of practice they want and create a practice that is a source of pride for them and their staff.

Retirement Plans for Physicians and Their Employees 309
Joel M. Blau

In the past, urologists planned for retirement by reviewing a potentially expansive list of income sources, such as social security, pensions from health care organizations, and income from investment portfolios. Today, planning for retirement is more focused on areas that physicians are able to control and to which they can contribute. For example, now it is appropriate to question whether or not social security will be available for retirement income. It is becoming more important to plan well in advance for the income needs that will exist during retirement.

GOAL STATEMENT

The goal of *Urologic Clinics of North America* is to keep practicing urologists and urology residents up to date with current clinical practice in urology by providing timely articles reviewing the state of the art in patient care.

ACCREDITATION

The *Urologic Clinics of North America* is planned and implemented in accordance with the Essential Areas and Policies of the Accreditation Council for Continuing Medical Education (ACCME) through the joint sponsorship of the University of Virginia School of Medicine and Elsevier. The University of Virginia School of Medicine is accredited by the ACCME to provide continuing medical education for physicians.

The University of Virginia School of Medicine designates this educational activity for a maximum of 60 category 1 credits per year, 15 category 1 credits per issue, toward the AMA Physician's Recognition Award. Each physician should claim only those credits that he/she actually spent in the activity.

The American Medical Association has determined that physicians not licensed in the US who participate in this CME activity are eligible for AMA PRA category 1 credit.

Category 1 credit can be earned by reading the text material, taking the CME examination online at http://www.theclinics.com/home/cme, and completing the evaluation. After taking the test, you will be required to review any and all incorrect answers. Following completion of the test and evaluation, your credit will be awarded and you may print your certificate.

FACULTY DISCLOSURE

As a provider accredited by the Accreditation Council for Continuing Medical Education (ACCME), the Office of Continuing Medical Education of the University of Virginia School of Medicine must ensure balance, independence, objectivity, and scientific rigor in all its individually sponsored or jointly sponsored educational activities. All authors/editors participating in a sponsored activity are expected to disclose to the readers any significant financial interest or other relationship (1) with the manufacturer(s) of any commercial product(s) and/or provider(s) of commercial services discussed in an educational presentation and (2) with any commercial supporters of the activity (significant financial interest or other relationship can include such things as grants or research support, employee, consultant, stock holder, member of speakers bureau, etc.) The intent of this disclosure is not to prevent authors/editors with a significant financial or other relationship from writing an article, but rather to provide readers with information on which they can make their own judgments. It remains for the readers to determine whether the author's/editor's interest or relationships may influence the article with regard to exposition or conclusion.

The authors/editors listed below have identified no professional or financial affiliations related to their presentation:
Joseph W. Akornor, MD; Fatih Atug, MD; Neil Baum, MD; Catherine Bewick, Acquisitions Editor; Joel M. Blau, CFP; Erik P. Castle, MD; Emily E. Cole, MD; Roger R. Dmochowski, MD, FACS; Vikram S. Dogra, MD; Nick A. Fabrizio, PhD, FACMPE, FACHE; Kenneth T. Hertz, CMPE; Paulita A. Keith, CPA; Sarah E. McAchran, MD; Ayay Nehra, MD; Martin I. Resnick, MD and Consulting Editor; Richard Rutherford, CMPE; Joseph W. Segura, MD; Stephanie N. Stinchcomb, CPC, CCS-P; and, Raju Thomas, MD, FACS, MHA.

Disclosure of Discussion of non-FDA approved uses for pharmaceutical products and/or medical devices: The University of Virginia School of Medicine, as an ACCME provider, requires that all faculty presenters identify and disclose any "off label" uses for pharmaceutical and medical device products. The University of Virginia School of Medicine recommends that each physician fully review all the available data on new products or procedures prior to instituting them with patients.

The authors who provided disclosure will NOT be discussing the off-label use of any pharmaceutical or medical device product.

The authors/editors listed below have not provided disclosure or off-label information:
David M. Andrew, JD; William F. Gee, MD, Guest Editor; and Cindy Spears.

TO ENROLL

To enroll in the *Urologic Clinics of North America* Continuing Medical Education program, call customer service at 1-800-654-2452 or visit us online at www.theclinics.com/home/cme. The CME program is available to subscribers for an additional fee of $165.00.

FORTHCOMING ISSUES

THE CLINICS ARE NOW AVAILABLE ONLINE!

Access your subscription at:
http://www.theclinics.com

UROLOGIC CLINICS of North America

Urol Clin N Am 32 (2005) xi

Foreword

Office Management and Procedures

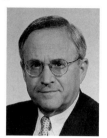

Martin I. Resnick, MD
Consulting Editor

Two decades ago, urologic office practice was primarily directed at managing relatively simple urologic disorders such as urinary tract infection and prostatitis and also in preparing patients for either further diagnostic studies or therapeutic procedures. Most urologists found that monies generated from this activity most typically covered the expense of running an office. Today, office practice has evolved to not only providing an environment for both diagnostic and therapeutic procedures but also has become a significant source of personal income to practicing urologists.

Dr. Gee has clearly selected topics and authors emphasizing this change in practice activity. The topics addressed vary from the importance of practice management to application of diagnostic procedures. All are important, and all urologists—whether in private practice or in an academic environment—need to be aware of these activities. Without a doubt, all should be interested in this important issue.

Martin I. Resnick, MD
Lester Persky Professor and Chairman
Department of Urology
Case Western Reserve University
School of Medicine/University Hospitals
11100 Euclid Avenue
Cleveland, OH 44106, USA

E-mail address: martin.resnick@case.edu

0094-0143/05/$ - see front matter © 2005 Elsevier Inc. All rights reserved.
doi:10.1016/j.ucl.2005.04.001

ELSEVIER
SAUNDERS

Urol Clin N Am 32 (2005) xiii

UROLOGIC
CLINICS
of North America

Preface

Office Management and Procedures

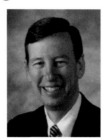

William F. Gee, MD
Guest Editor

Twenty-five years ago, the *Urologic Clinics of North America* published an issue entitled "Office Urology." That issue dealt with the clinical aspects of the office from performing urine cultures to treating male sexual dysfunction. In 1980 there were no lithotriptors, no ureteroscopes, no lasers, no microwaves, no laparoscopes, no robots, no decent ultrasound, no PSA, and no drugs that really worked to treat erectile dysfunction. How times have changed.

This issue is intended to address the complex challenges of office management and the many issues in this area that did not exist in 1980.

Proper office management has become a complex and vital component of the successful medical practice in the twenty-first century. Ever-shrinking reimbursement, more and more rules and regulations, and increasing intrusion by governmental entities mandate a thorough understanding of these issues. Whether you are in solo practice, a single-specialty urology group, a multi-specialty group, or an academic medical center, you are no longer immune from these issues—they affect us all, regardless of where we practice. In my search for authors in various areas of practice management, I came across some incredibly knowledgeable individuals who were willing to put their expertise down on paper. I think you will find these articles not only informative but of real practical use in running your practice.

The issue concludes with four outstanding articles on many of the procedures we perform most commonly in our offices, including ultrasound, urodynamics, various endoscopic procedures, treatment of benign genital lesions, and in-office treatment of BPH.

Two areas that were not addressed are the office laboratory and office radiologic imaging, other than ultrasound. Many larger urology practices have sophisticated laboratory chemistry processing devices and are developing in-office pathology for processing prostate biopsy and other specimens. In addition, several urology practices are installing CT scanners and other advanced and sophisticated imaging devices. Many of these ventures involve unique individual state laws, "certificates of need," and complex federal regulations. Suffice it to say that many urology practices are delving into these areas with considerable success, being ever mindful to seek competent legal advice before proceeding.

William F. Gee, MD
Commonwealth Urology
1760 Nicholasville Road
Lexington, KY 40503, USA

E-mail address: w.f.gee@att.net

0094-0143/05/$ - see front matter © 2005 Elsevier Inc. All rights reserved.
doi:10.1016/j.ucl.2005.04.005

ELSEVIER
SAUNDERS

Urol Clin N Am 32 (2005) 253–262

UROLOGIC
CLINICS
of North America

Office Management: Personnel Issues Overview

David M. Andrew, JD

Hemmer Pangburn DeFrank PLLC, 250 Grandview Drive,
Suite 200, Ft. Mitchell, KY 41017, USA

Employers continue to face an increasing number of personnel issues in managing medical practices. Because of the personnel issues and the ever-present effect they can have on a medical practice, this article addresses personnel issues faced by many employers, including medical practices.

Although it is impossible to address in detail all personnel concerns that could affect a medical practice, the information provided deals with the most common or frequent problems faced by employers. This article addresses basic background information relating to the most common and frequent problems faced by employers, including

- The Family and Medical Leave Act
- The Americans with Disabilities Act (ADA)
- The Civil Rights Act of 1964
- The Age Discrimination in Employment Act (ADEA)

This article also addresses basic methods that employers can use to avoid or effectively deal with personnel issues when they arise, including employee handbooks, investigations of claims, and termination of employees.

Although this article is not exhaustive and should not be relied on for any specific personnel issues that employers may face, it does provide basic information relating to personnel matters and related concerns.

Family and Medical Leave Act

Purpose

The Family and Medical Leave Act is an attempt to allow employees to have more time

E-mail address: Dandrew@Hemmerlaw.com

with their families under warranted circumstances. "The act is intended to balance the demands of the work place with the needs of families, and to promote national interests in preserving family integrity" [1]. By providing assurances to family members and employers that employees can address family issues with some job security, it was Congress' intent to benefit employers and employees with a productive and stable work environment [2].

Affected employer

The Family and Medical Leave Act applies to employers that employ at least 50 or more employees each working day during each of 20 or more calendar workweeks in the current or preceding calendar year within a 75-mile radius [3]. When determining if an employer has 50 or more employees, the term "employee," for the purposes of the Family and Medical Leave Act, is taken from the Fair Labor Standards Act [4]. This definition is broader than a simple master-servant relationship. The courts have stated that there is no one definition that solves all problems and limitations of the employer-employee relationship under the Family and Medical Leave Act and that a determination of the relationship cannot be based on isolated factors but depends on the entire set of circumstances surrounding employment relationships [5].

Included in the definition of employer is the idea of joint employment. Joint employment is when two or more businesses exercise some control over the work or work conditions of employees. Under these circumstances, a business may be a joint employer for purposes of the Family and Medical Leave Act. For example, the regulations specifically address the issue of leased employees. "For example, an employer who

0094-0143/05/$ - see front matter © 2005 Elsevier Inc. All rights reserved.
doi:10.1016/j.ucl.2005.03.008

jointly employs 15 workers from a leasing or temporary help agency and 40 workers is covered by FMLA" [6]. Based on this description, employers are the primary employer for permanent workers and the secondary employer for the leased employees. Nevertheless, both sets of employees must be counted for purposes of establishing if an employer is subject to the provisions of the Family and Medical Leave Act.

Notice

Employers subject to the requirements of the Family and Medical Leave Act must post a notice summarizing the Family and Medical Leave Act's important provisions and the procedures for filing a charge with the Department of Labor Wage and Hour Division for an employer violation of the act. The notice must be posted in a conspicuous place on the premises, where it can be seen easily by employees and applicants [7].

If employers provide their employees with an employee handbook or other written guidance concerning employee rights, information concerning employee rights and obligations under the Family and Medical Leave Act must be included in the document [8].

Eligibility

Not all employees are entitled to leave under the Family and Medical Leave Act. The law sets minimum lengths of service and hours of work requirements that employees must satisfy. Before employees become eligible for leave under the Family and Medical Leave Act, they must have been employed by the same employer for at least 12 months and must have worked at least 1250 hours during the 12 months preceding the leave. The Family and Medical Leave Act states that the 12 months of employment do not need to be consecutive [9].

Reason for leave

The Family and Medical Leave Act provides up to 12 weeks per year of unpaid leave to eligible employees and requires employers to restore those employees to the same or equivalent position upon their return. The Family and Medical Leave Act allows for specific circumstances and how or when leave must be taken. The Family and Medical Leave Act allows for eligible employees (male or female) to take leave for (1) the birth and care of a newborn child; (2) the adoption or placement in foster care of a child; and (3) the care of a seriously ill child, spouse, or parent or the employee's own serious illness.

Serious health conditions

Serious health conditions entitling employees to time away from work pursuant to the Family and Medical Leave Act include, but are not limited to

- Inpatient care in a hospital, hospice, or residential medical care facility; any period of incapacity; or any subsequent treatment [10]
- Continuing treatment by a health care provider after a period of incapacity (inability to work, attend school, or perform other regular activities as a result of the serious health condition, treatment, or recovery) of more than 3 consecutive calendar days and any subsequent treatment [11]
- Period of incapacity as a result of pregnancy or prenatal care [12]
- A chronic serious health condition [13]
- A period of incapacity that is permanent or long term for which treatment may not be effective (Alzheimer's, stroke, or terminal diseases) [14]

Employee duties

Employees must provide employers 30 days advanced notice of the need for foreseeable leave because of an expected birth, placement of a child for adoption or foster care, or planned medical treatment of a serious condition of the employee or family member [15]. If earlier notice is not practicable, or the need for leave is not foreseeable, notice must be given as soon as is practicable. It is expected that notice be given within 1 or 2 working days [16]. Notice should be given in person, by telephone, or by electronic method. Employees are not required to request Family and Medical Leave specifically by name to have leave started [17].

Medical certification

If the leave request is based on an employee's own serious health condition or the serious health condition of an employee's family member, employers can require that the request be accompanied by certification from a health care provider. Employers can require any employee to obtain a second opinion (at the employer's expense) if the validity of the certification is in doubt. If the two opinions conflict, the employer may pay for a third opinion that must be approved jointly by the employer and the employee. The third opinion is final [18].

Employer duties

When employees provide notice of a need for leave, the Department of Labor requires employers to provide employees with notice describing the employees' obligations and explaining the consequences of a failure to meet the obligations. The notice should include information on the following:

- The leave counted against the employee's 12 weeks
- Medical certification requirements
- The employee's right to use paid leave and whether the employer does or does not require the substitution of paid leave
- Requirements concerning payment of health insurance
- Requirements for fitness of duty certificate before the employee's restoration to employment
- Where applicable, the employee's status as a key employee and the consequences thereof
- The employee's right to restoration to the same or equivalent job upon return from leave
- The employee's potential liability for payment of health insurance premiums paid by the employer during the unpaid leave if the employee fails to return to work after leave

Employers are responsible for designating leave, paid or unpaid, as Family and Medical Leave Act leave [19]. Even if employees do not request Family and Medical Leave Act leave, employers can designate it as such. If employers fail to designate a leave as Family and Medical Leave Act leave, employers may not be able to do so retroactively [20]. Current court cases state, however, that these types of restrictions on retroactive application of leave may act as a penalty to employers and may not prohibit retroactive application. Nevertheless, employers should abide by the notification provisions found within the Family and Medical Leave Act and inform employees of their rights under the Family and Medical Leave Act.

Amount of leave

Eligible employees are entitled to 12 workweeks of leave during any 12-month period for any Family and Medical Leave Act qualifying event [21].

To determine the 12-month period in which the leave entitlement occurs, employers can choose from (1) the calendar year, (2) any fixed 12-month leave year, (3) the 12-month period measured forward from the date of an employee's first leave, or (4) a rolling 12-month period measured backward from the date the employee used any leave [22]. Employers are allowed to choose any of the four methods for determining the 12-month period for leave; however, the method chosen by an employer must be applied consistently and uniformly to all employees. Moreover, employers who wish to change their method of calculating leave eligibility are required to give at least 60 days notice to all employees and the employees must retain their full 12 weeks of leave [23].

Types of leave

The Family and Medical Leave Act requires that leave may be taken on an intermittent or reduced leave schedule under certain circumstances. Intermittent leave is defined as taking separate blocks of time because of a single qualifying reason. A reduced leave schedule is a leave schedule that reduces an employee's usual number of working hours per workweek or hours per workday [24]. When leave is taken after the birth of a child or placement of a child for adoption or foster care, employees may take only intermittent leave or reduced leave if their employer agrees. The employer's agreement is not required, however, when a mother has a serious health condition in connection with the birth of a child or if a newborn child has a serious health condition [25].

Benefits during leave

Generally, Family and Medical Leave Act leave is unpaid; however, eligible employees are allowed to choose to substitute paid leave for unpaid leave. If employees do not choose to substitute paid leave, employers may require employees to use all accrued paid leave that they are entitled to before taking unpaid leave [26].

During any Family and Medical Leave Act leave, employers must maintain employees' coverage under any group health plan on the same conditions as coverage would have been provided if employees had been employed continuously during the entire leave period [27]. Any shared group health plans, however, that were paid for by employees before their leave must continue to be paid by the employee during the period of leave [28].

Any employees who take leave are not entitled to the accrual of additional benefits or seniority that may occur during the period of unpaid leave [29]. Leaves shall not be counted or treated as breaks in services for purposes of vesting or eligibility to participate in retirement plans. Furthermore, time taken away from work as Family and Medical Leave Act leave need not be treated as credited services for purposes of benefit accrual, vesting, and eligibility to participate [30].

Employees' rights upon returning from leave

Upon return from leave, employees are entitled to return to the same position they held when leave commenced or to an equivalent position with equivalent benefits, pay, and other terms and conditions of employment [31].

An equivalent position is one that is virtually identical to the former position in terms of pay, benefits, and work conditions, including privileges and status. It must involve the same or similar duties and responsibilities [32].

Americans with Disability Act

Purpose

The United States Congress found that, historically, society tended to isolate and segregate individuals who had disabilities and that discrimination against those individuals who had disabilities persisted in multiple sectors of society. The United States Congress found that individuals who had disabilities had no legal recourse to address discrimination. To rectify the situation, Congress enacted the ADA in 1990. The purpose of the ADA was to provide a national mandate for the elimination of discrimination against individuals who have disabilities by providing standards governing the treatment of said individuals [33]. The ADA applies to employers with 15 or more employees for each of the 20 or more calendar weeks in the current or preceding year [34].

Disability

The ADA defines disability as

1. A physical or mental impairment that substantially limits one or more of the major life actions of such individual

2. A record of such an impairment
3. Being regarded as having such an impairment [35]

In the ADA, Congress attempts to define the pertinent sections and clauses to determine disability. The Courts, however, have taken up the determination of what constitutes a disability under the ADA.

Recent cases have attempted to define what constitutes a disability for purposes of the ADA. In *Toyota Manufacturing, Ky. Inc. v. Williams* [36], the Court established several factors to assist in determining if individuals are disabled:

- The ADA allows a person to establish disability if the condition affects any major life function, not simply functions related to work.
- An employee does not have to prove that the impairment limits an entire class of activities.
- Any analysis of the ADA needs to determine how the condition affects not only the ability to do a job but also the ability to perform daily activities.
- The determination of disability relies not only on medical evidence but also an analysis has to be undertaken as to how those restrictions or conditions affect the work and daily activities of the employee.

Recently, the United States Supreme Court also dealt with corrective measures as mitigating circumstances when determining if individuals are disabled. In *Sutton v. United Airlines, Inc.*, the Court found that individuals who have corrective measures, including medications or appliances, that control an alleged disability are not disabilities for ADA purposes [37].

Even though mitigating measures may eliminate individuals from being disabled for ADA purposes, claims of disability must be assessed on an individual basis. In some circumstances, the mitigating circumstance may have side effects or other factors that still cause individuals to be disabled.

In addition to employees claiming to be disabled, employees can have a record of impairment or be treated as being disabled. *A record of impairment* means that individuals have a history of, or have been misclassified as having, a mental or physical impairment that substantially limits one or more major life activities [38].

Also, if employers regard individuals as having impairment, then individuals can be determined as having a disability. *Is regarded as having such an impairment* means

1. Has a physical or mental impairment that does not limit major life activities substantially but is treated by a covered entity as constituting such limitations
2. Has a physical and mental impairment that limits major life activities substantially only as a result of the attitudes of others toward such impairment
3. Has none of the impairments defined in paragraph (h)(1) or (2) of this section but is treated by covered entity as having a substantially limiting impairment [39].

The attitudes and treatment of employees by employers can qualify individuals as having a disability for ADA purposes. Therefore, employers need to take caution in treating individuals who have any impairment that could be considered a disability.

Medical examinations

Employers may not require a pre-employment examination or inquire into individual health histories before an offer of employment. The only acceptable pre-employment inquiry is whether or not the applicant is capable of performing the job-related functions [40]. After an offer of employment is made and before the commencement of the employment duties and as a condition to the offer of employment, examinations may be undertaken if

1. All similarly situated employees are subject to the examination
2. The information regarding the medical condition or history is maintained properly away from other information
3. The results of the examination are used only in conjunction with the ADA [41].

Individuals who have disabilities and their job functions

Qualified individuals who have a disability means individuals who have a disability and who satisfy the requisite skill, experience, education, and other job-related requirements of the employment position such individual holds or desires, and who, with or without reasonable accommodation, can perform the essential functions of such position [42].

Reasonable accommodation means

1. Modifications or adjustments to a job application process that enable a qualified applicant who has a disability to be considered for the position such qualified applicant desires; or
2. Modifications or adjustments to the work environment or to the manner or circumstances under which the position however desired is customarily performed that enable qualified individuals who have a disability to perform the essential functions of that position; or
3. Modifications or adjustments that enable a covered entity employee who has a disability to enjoy equal benefits and privileges of employment as are enjoyed by its other similarly situated employees who do not disabilities [43]

Reasonable accommodations may include but are not limited to

- Making existing facilities accessible to individuals who have disabilities
- Job restructuring
- Part-time or modified work schedules
- Reassignment to vacant positions
- Acquisition of modifications of equipment or devices
- Training materials or policies
- Provisions of qualified readers or interpreters
- Other accommodations for individuals who have disabilities [44]

Employers must provide accommodations to employees who have disabilities, unless to do so creates an undue hardship on employers. To determine if undue hardship exists, the following factors are to be considered:

- The nature and net cost of the accommodation
- The overall financial resources of the facility or facilities
- The overall financial resources of the employer
- The type of operation or operations of the employer
- The impact of the accommodation on the operation of the facility
- The fact that substantial significant risks of substantial harm to the health or safety of the individual cannot be limited or reduced by reasonable accommodation [45]

Civil Rights Act of 1964

Purpose

Title VII of the Civil Rights Act of 1964 applies to employers who have 15 or more employees for each working day in each of the 20 or more calendar weeks in the current or preceding calendar year [46]. The Civil Rights Act makes it unlawful for employers to

1. Fail or refuse to hire or to discharge individuals, or otherwise discriminate against individuals, with respect to compensation, terms, conditions, or privileges of employment, because of individuals' race, color, religion, sex, or national origin
2. Limit, segregate, or classify employees or applicants for employment in a way which would deprive or tend to deprive individuals of employment opportunities or otherwise adversely affect their status as employees, because of such individuals' race, color, religion, sex, or national origin [47]

Application

In order for employees to prove a violation of the Civil Rights Act, the complaining party must demonstrate that he or she was part of a protected class and that the employer's actions caused disparate impact on the basis of race, color, religion, sex, or national origin. At that time, the employers have the opportunity to show or demonstrate that the employment practice is job related and based on a business necessity [48].

Age Discrimination in Employment Act

Purpose

The United States Congress determined that older workers found themselves at a disadvantage in efforts to retain employment and regain employment when displaced from jobs. Therefore, it was the purpose of the ADEA to promote employment of older persons based on ability rather than age, to prohibit age discrimination, and to help employers and workers find ways of resolving problems arising from the impact of age on employment [49].

The ADEA applies to employers that have 20 or more employees for each working day and each of the 20 or more calendar weeks in the current or proceeding calendar year [50]. The ADEA makes it unlawful for employers to

1. Fail or refuse to hire or to discharge individuals or otherwise discriminate against individuals with respect to his compensation, terms, conditions, or privileges of employment, because of such individual's age
2. Limit, segregate, or classify employees in any way that would deprive or tend to deprive any individuals of employment opportunities or otherwise adversely affect their status as an employee, because of such individual's age
3. Reduce the wage rate of any employee to comply with this chapter [51]

Application

The ADEA applies only to individuals who are at least 40 years of age [52]. The ADEA does not apply, however, in a situation in which bona fide executives or high policymaking individuals are forced into compulsory retirement at the age 65. In order for the exemption to apply, employees must

1. Obtain 65 years of age
2. For the 2-year period immediately before retirement, be employed in a bona fide executive or high policymaking position
3. Be entitled to an immediate nonforfeitable annual retirement benefit from the company pension, profit-sharing, savings, or deferred compensation plan or any combination of such plans
4. The plan or plans equals, in the aggregate, at least $44,000 [53]

Handling personnel issues

Employee handbooks

Today, most employers provide employee handbooks to their employees. Employee handbooks typically contain rules, regulations, and office procedures for particular employers. Although employers have different rules and regulations and different laws govern different states of employment, employee handbooks should contain some basic information applicable to all employers.

Every handbook should contain a disclaimer that the employee handbook is being provided only for informational purposes and its contents should not be interpreted as a contract between employers and the employees. Along with a disclaimer regarding an employment contract, a disclaimer should state that the contents of the handbook cannot be changed except by written agreement of a person in a management position who has authority to make such changes. This disclaimer simply avoids employees stating that lower supervisors or managers allowed employees to change specific aspects of the employee handbook. This allows for consistency in the application of the handbook.

If applicable, the Family and Medical Leave Act disclosure should be contained in the handbook, as required by the Family and Medical Leave Act.

Issues of employment discrimination, in any manner, should be addressed. Employees should be aware that if perceived discrimination in any form occurs, it is the employees' responsibility to report the behavior to management as soon as possible. A reporting chain of command should be provided in the event that an employee's direct manager allegedly is committing the misconduct. Employees should be assured that all complaints are taken seriously and an immediate, full, and confidential investigation conducted. Employees should be informed that no remedial action will be taken against reporting employees and that, after an appropriate investigation, necessary actions will be taken against the alleged offending party.

Employee handbooks also should address basic benefits, including time off, company policies, and benefits. It is easier to deal with the issues up front rather than have employees asking about these issues when they arise.

Issues regarding disciplinary procedures and actions should be included. If disciplinary procedures for employees are set forth in a handbook, then employers should be consistent when handling disciplinary matters. Employers cannot pick and choose to enforce disciplinary procedures based on whether or not employees are good or bad. When dealing with disciplinary matters, consistency and fair application are required. When employers make exceptions for perceived good employees, problems arise. Exceptions make it difficult for employers to show consistency in disciplinary matters and, therefore, expose potential employment issues.

Investigations

During the course of employment, invariably an employee raises personnel issues relating to harassment, discrimination, or some other type of alleged misconduct. At that time, employers must conduct a fair and reasonable investigation into an allegation. Employers must inform employees that there will be no retaliation and that complaints kept confidential.

Employment investigations need to be conducted by an unbiased individual who is least likely affected by the investigation to insure that investigations are conducted in a fair and reasonable manner.

A thorough interview with a complaining employee should be conducted as soon as possible. All information relating to the alleged act or actions should be documented, including time, place, and individuals involved. Employers should gain as much information as possible. Employees should have an opportunity to reflect on the interview and at a later, but contemporaneous, time period, provide any additional information.

Once the information and pertinent facts are gathered, the investigation must take place. The investigation includes

1. Interviewing the individual involved with the alleged conduct
2. Interviewing any potential witnesses
3. Interviewing any and all individuals who may have any information regarding the alleged conduct, including prior complaints or issues
4. Reviewing any and all information available relating to the alleged incident
5. Reviewing any and all relevant materials relating to the alleged conduct
6. Reviewing all information

Once the investigation is complete, it is necessary to determine if the alleged conduct did or did not take place and whether or not any remedial action will be taken. At that time, the complaining employee should be addressed again and informed of the results of the investigation, including what action, if any, will be taken as a result of the investigation.

By conducting a proper investigation and taking appropriate, if any, remedial action, employers have an opportunity to insulate themselves from any potential liability. In recent United States Supreme Court cases, the Court determined that employers that take reasonable measures to protect employees against sexual harassment are provided an affirmative defense against claims brought by those employees. Reasonable actions should be taken before any alleged claim by informing all employees that any type of discriminatory action, sexual or otherwise, is prohibited. Employees need to be informed of the proper process for reporting alleged claims. Moreover, once a complaint is made, by conducting a reasonable and thorough investigation and taking the appropriate remedial action, employers show that they take reasonable measures to protect employees.

Although the Supreme Court cases dealt with sexual harassment, it is a good policy to follow the advice of the Court in similarly situated circumstances. Therefore, it benefits employers to inform all employees that any discriminatory conduct is not tolerated and of the potential repercussions for participating in discriminatory conduct. Moreover, reasonable and thorough investigations may limit any liability as a result of alleged discriminatory conduct.

Again, consistency is vital when addressing any personnel issue, including discriminatory conduct. If employers consistently address and take action relating to any alleged conduct, regardless of the alleged actor, then employers help insulate themselves from liability. Too often, employers do not enforce their own policies and, therefore, open themselves up to liability.

Employee termination

Eventually, most employers have to terminate an employee and be faced with potential issues related to a wrongful termination. To guard or minimize a wrongful termination claim, an analysis should be undertaken by employers before terminating an employee. Before terminating an employee, employers should review the following:

- Is the employee being terminated for verifiable work-related reasons, such as
  - Absenteeism
  - Tardiness
  - Insubordination
  - Failure to follow employer rules
  - Poor performance
- If an employee is being terminated for verifiable work-related reasons, has the employer
  - Followed its own disciplinary procedures as set forth in the employee handbook or followed procedures consistently used in the past
  - Documented appropriately the reasons for the verifiable work-related termination

- Consistently enforced similar rules and regulations with other employees

After employers have conducted an analysis of whether or not there are verifiable work-related reasons for terminating an employee, employers should evaluate if there are non–work-related issues that could give rise to a potential discriminatory claim. These factors include

- Race
- Age (over 40)
- Nationality
- Sex
- Religion
- Prior complaints of harassment or discrimination
- Inconsistent application of rules or regulations
- Other non–work-related issues

Non–work-related issues, although they do not prevent termination, may raise red flags in the event issues are raised by the terminated employee at a later date. If employers are consistent in application of rules and procedures for job performance, however, the non–work-related issues should not prevent termination.

Once they decide to terminate an employee, employers are faced with how to terminate an employee. The question of how to terminate an employee involves the following issues:

- Who terminates the employee
- How to terminate the employee, verbally or in writing
- When to terminate an employee
- Reason given to an employee for termination
- Offer of any compensation or attempt to obtain a release of claims

Individual states may address how to terminate or what procedures must be followed when terminating an employee. If no specifics regarding termination are dictated by state law, termination normally is conducted by someone in the human resources department or management of the practice. The termination can be either in writing or verbal depending on the practice of employers. The reason for termination should state the documented work reason that has been applied consistently by the employer.

When employees are terminated, they should gather their belongings and immediately leave the work site after turning over any access devices to the work site. Employers should insure that any electronic access to computers, voice mail, or other electronic equipment is terminated.

Upon termination, benefits owed to the employee typically are dictated by state law, including whether or not the employee receives accrued vacation or personal time. Employers can agree to a severance package over and above what is dictated by applicable law or can provide nothing other than what is required.

Employers can attempt to obtain a waiver for any potential claims employees may have against them. If employers decide to obtain a waiver, sufficient consideration should be given to warrant and justify the waiver.

If individuals are over 40, then any waiver must satisfy specific criteria as outlined in the Older Workers' Benefit Protection Act and adopted by ADEA. These requirements include

- The waiver is knowing and voluntary and written in a manner calculated to be understood by such individual or by the average individual eligible to participate.
- The waiver refers to the rights or claims arising under the ADEA.
- No waiver for rights or claims arising after the date of the waiver.
- There must be consideration for a separate and distinct value.
- The individual is advised in writing to consult with an attorney before executing the agreement.
- The individual is given a period of 21 days, at a minimum, to consider the agreement.
- The agreement provides that for a period of at least 7 days after execution, the individual can revoke the agreement [54].

Summary

Employers can protect themselves reasonably from personnel and employment issues by having a basic understanding of employment laws and regulations that affect their practice. Moreover, by applying the basic rules and procedures of the practice consistently and fairly, practices can protect and insulate themselves from potential employment-related issues.

This article is not intended as an all-inclusive guide to personnel and employment issues facing employers. It does provide, however, a basic understanding of some of the common issues experienced by employers and basic ways to protect themselves. Each individual employment situation contains its own specific set of facts and carries its own specific risks. Therefore, each must be addressed accordingly with an understanding of the laws and regulations that pertain to that particular situation.

References

[1] 29 C.F.R. §825.101(a).
[2] 29 C.F.R. §825.101(b).
[3] 29 C.F.R. §825.104(1).
[4] Fair Labor Standards Act, §3(g).
[5] 29 C.F.R. §825.105.
[6] 29 C.F.R. §825.160(d).
[7] 29 C.F.R. §825.300.
[8] 29 C.F.R. §825.301 (a)(9).
[9] 29 C.F.R. §825.111.
[10] 29 C.F.R. §825.114(1).
[11] 29 C.F.R. §825.114(2)(i).
[12] 29 C.F.R. §825.114(11).
[13] 29 C.F.R. §825.164(2)(iii).
[14] 29 C.F.R. §825.114(2)(iv).
[15] 29 C.R.F. §825.302(a).
[16] 29 C.F.R. §825.303(a).
[17] 29 C.F.R. §825.303(6).
[18] 29 C.F.R. §825.305, 308.
[19] 20 C.F.R. §825(a)(2).
[20] 20 C.F.R. §825.208(e)(1).
[21] 29 C.F.R. §825.200(a).
[22] 29 C.F.R. §825.200(b)(1–4).
[23] 29 C.F.R. §825.200(d)(1).
[24] 29 C.F.R. §825.203(a).
[25] 29 C.F.R. §825.203(b).
[26] 29 C.F.R. §825.207(a).
[27] 29 C.F.R. §825.209(a).
[28] 29 C.F.R. §825.210(a).
[29] 29 C.F.R. §825.215(d)(2).
[30] 29 C.F.R. §825.215.
[31] 29 C.F.R. §825.214.
[32] 29 C.F.R. §825.215.
[33] 42 C.F.R. 12101(a) and (b).
[34] 29 C.F.R. §1630.2(e).
[35] 29 C.F.R. 1630.2(g)(1–3).
[36] *Toyota Manufacturing, Ky. Inc. v. Williams*, 535 US 184 (January 2002).
[37] *Sutton v. United Airlines, Inc.*, 527 US 471 (June 1999).
[38] 29 C.F.R. 1630.2(k).
[39] 29 C.F.R. 1630.2(l).
[40] 42 U.S.C. 12112(d)(2).
[41] 42 U.S.C. §12112(d)(3).
[42] 29 C.F.R. §1630.2(m).
[43] 29 C.F.R. §1630.2(o)(1).
[44] 29 C.F.R. §1630.2(2)(O)(i) and (ii).
[45] 29 C.F.R. §1630.2(p–r).
[46] 42 U.S.C. §2000e(b).

[47] 42 U.S.C. §2000e–2, (a)(1) and (2).

[48] 42 U.S.C. §2000e–2(k).

[49] 29 U.S.C. §621(a) and (b).

[50] 29 U.S.C. §630(b).

[51] 29 U.S.C. §623(a)(1–3).

[52] 29 U.S.C. §631(a).

[53] 29 U.S.C. §631(c)(1).

[54] 29 U.S.C. §626(f).

ELSEVIER
SAUNDERS

Urol Clin N Am 32 (2005) 263–269

UROLOGIC
CLINICS
of North America

The Role of the Accountant in Your Practice

Paulita A. Keith, CPA

Healthcare Practice Consultants, LLC, 920 Dupont Road, Suite 200, Louisville, KY 40207, USA

A business accountant should be a trusted business advisor and not-so-silent partner. Accountants can assist in making the ordinary everyday decisions in a practice, such as type of business entity under which to operate; type of compensation model a practice should use; type of funding strategy that should be used for capital improvements (eg, leasing versus buying); depreciation methods that should be used; tax strategies for maximizing deductions; retirement plan strategies; practice growth strategies; and many other practice decisions.

Choice of business entity

The choice of business entity is important for every practice. Each business entity has its own legal and tax implications, which, of course, vary from state to state. Some of the basic elements of each type of entity are:

Sole proprietor

- One owner
- Reports income and loss on Schedule C
- Owner pays income tax
- No liability protection

Partnership

- Two or more owners
- Reports income and loss on Form 1065 with K-1s showing each owner's share of income and deductions
- Owners pay income tax
- Must have basis to deduct losses
- Cannot deduct partner fringe benefits, such as health insurance, disability insurance, long-term care insurance, and group term life insurance, although may be able to deduct health insurance and long-term care insurance on personal return
- No liability protection

Limited liability company and limited liability partnership

- Number of owners depends on state law
- A limited liability company (LLC) and a limited liability partnership (LLP) are not specific entities for tax purposes, meaning that there is not an LLC or LLP tax return. An LLC or LLP must elect the entity it wishes to be for tax purposes. If no election is made, a single-member LLC defaults to a disregarded entity and is treated as a sole proprietorship, and an LLC or LLP with more than one member defaults to a partnership.
- Reporting of income and loss depends on entity election
- Payment of income taxes depends on entity election
- Limited liability protection
- LLC and LLP laws depend on the state in which they are organized. Some states allow for single-member LLCs and some do not.

C corporation

- One or more owners
- Reports income and loss on Form 1120
- Entity pays income taxes
- Potential for double taxation
- Disability premiums paid through corporation for owners are deductible but, if disability is paid under policy, proceeds are taxable
- Some liability protection

E-mail address: hpcllc@bellsouth.net

0094-0143/05/$ - see front matter © 2005 Elsevier Inc. All rights reserved.
doi:10.1016/j.ucl.2005.03.011

urologic.theclinics.com

S corporation

- One to 100 owners
- Reports income and loss on Form 1120S with K-1s showing each owner's share of income and deductions
- Owners pay income tax
- Must have basis to deduct losses
- Two percent of owners must include fringe benefits in taxable income, although may be able to deduct health insurance and long-term care insurance on personal tax return
- Some liability protection

Practice compensation models

Equitably distributing practice income among a practice's physicians always is a challenge. In creating a compensation model, the physicians first must agree, in concept, to the formula and the theory behind it. Furthermore, the less complicated a group's formula is, the easier it is to substantiate, explain it to potential partners entering a practice, and, obviously, calculate. Entire books are written illustrating compensation calculations. Some of the common approaches are discussed in this article.

Compensation divided equally

Under this formula, each member gets the same share of the profits. The advantage to this approach is that it is simplistic and can work well in groups in which the physicians are comparable producers. This approach generally does not work in groups in which physicians work at different paces. The disadvantage is that it does not provide an incentive to physicians to work harder and more efficiently.

Productivity

Under this formula, each group member gets a percentage of the group's profit based on the percentage of gross billings for that physician within the total physician gross billings for the group. The advantage to this approach is that it gives incentive to work harder and more efficiently and it accommodates producers at both ends of the spectrum. The disadvantage to this approach is that it may prompt physicians to compete for patients. Computation may be complex depending on the factors used. If the productivity formula is used, it must omit any division of Medicare- and Medicaid-designated health services as outlined in Stark laws.

Physician compensation based on productivity should have a method of dividing expenses, as appropriate, among the physicians. Fixed expenses that do not change according to productivity, such as rent, advertising, telephone, salaries, and benefits for shared office staff, should be divided equally. Variable expenses that productivity has a direct impacted on, such as medical supplies, equipment maintenance, and office supplies, should be divided based on productivity. Direct physician expenses that are specific to a physician, such as automobile expenses; dues; publications; licenses; continuing medical education; malpractice premiums; health, life, and disability insurances; and any staff working only with that physician, should be assigned to individual physicians.

This system allows physicians to have some flexibility in structuring their compensation packages. It enables physicians to spend *their* money between salary and fringe benefits while encouraging doctors to be cost conscious with a practice's money.

Part equal, part productivity

This compensation model is a combination of the equal and productivity formulas. It splits an agreed-upon percentage of the income equally among the physicians. The remaining percentage is split based on productivity.

Again, the productivity portion must omit any division of Medicare- and Medicaid-designated health services as outlined in Stark laws.

Base salary plus incentive

Under this formula, each physician is paid the same base compensation. Profits exceeding base compensation are divided as incentive compensation. Incentive compensation is based on a formula, such as charges, number of patient encounters, collections, and so forth. The advantage to this model is that it acknowledges that each physician contributes to the group and ensures a known salary. The disadvantage to this formula is that it may be a disincentive for producers. Furthermore, if the incentive is based on a type of productivity or volume, the formula must omit any Medicare- and Medicaid-designated health services as outlined in Stark laws.

When devising a compensation formula for a group, it is important to compensate the physicians fairly and equitably using only available cash. Formulas driven by a profit number on a financial statement often place the group in a cash-flow crunch because accounting profit generally does not correspond to available cash.

Capital improvements

Practices making investments in capital assets are faced with many options. Practices can lease equipment under a capital or operating lease, purchase assets outright, or finance equipment purchases through a bank loan. Costs should be analyzed to determine total out-of-pocket cash under each particular method. Tax ramifications also should be considered. Operating leases are deductible for tax purposes as payments are made. Operating leases include a provision that the leased asset may be purchased at the end of the term at fair market value. Capital leases are treated as an asset purchase. Assets that are purchased and placed in service during the year are subject to depreciation rules (discussed later). Capital leases contain a provision that the leased asset may be purchased for a nominal amount, usually $1.00, at the end of the lease term. For tax purposes, capital leases are treated the same as outright purchases or bank financed purchases.

When analyzing leases, it is important to consider the cash outlay of the entire transaction, including financing cost and tax savings. This approach enables practices to make the most educated decision when making investments in capital assets.

Depreciation methods

Depreciation is the method by which practices are allowed to deduct capital expenditures. Depreciation rules apply to most types of tangible and real property with the exception of land, which cannot be depreciated. It also applies to certain intangible property. Property to be depreciated includes buildings, machinery, vehicles, furniture, equipment, patents, copyrights, and computer software. To be depreciable, property must be owned by a practice, be used actively in a practice, have a determinable useful life, and be expected to last more than 1 year.

Depreciation expense begins in the year the property is placed in service and ends either in the year in which the cost has been recovered fully or

in the year in which the asset is disposed of—scrapped, sold, or otherwise taken out of service.

The basis of the property that is allowed to be depreciated under tax law is the cost multiplied by the percentage of business use.

The type of business property dictates the number of years over which property must be depreciated. Computers, typewriters, calculators, copiers, and high-tech medical equipment are depreciated over 5 years. Automobiles are deemed to be 5-year property but have special rules, which make the deduction different for them than from other 5-year properties. Office furniture and equipment, medical equipment, and any property that does not have a designated class life under the regulations are depreciated over 7 years. Improvements made directly to land, such as fences, roads, sidewalks, and parking lots, are depreciated over 15 years. Office buildings and leasehold improvements are depreciated over 39 years. (Because it takes 39 years to depreciate leasehold improvements, it is tax smart to have the landlord, if possible, pay for the improvements and add the cost to the rent.)

The date placed in service determines the convention that must be used in computing depreciation. Property placed in service under the midmonth convention, nonresidential real property, is deemed to be placed in service at the midpoint of the month. This means that half-month depreciation is allowed for the month in which the property was placed in service. If 40% of the total depreciable assets are placed in service in the last 3 months of the year, the midquarter convention applies. This means that all property placed in service in any quarter of the tax year is deemed placed in service at the midpoint of the quarter. If neither the midmonth or midquarter convention applies, the property is considered to be placed in service under the half-year convention. Under this convention, all property placed in service is treated as being placed in service at the midpoint of the year. This means that half-year of depreciation is allowed.

Property is depreciated under the Modified Accelerated Cost Recovery System (MACRS) method of depreciation. MACRS provides for three methods of depreciation: (1) the 200% declining balance method; (2) the 150% declining balance method; and (3) the straight-line method. The type of property dictates the method that must be used. Taxpayers may elect to use a different method of depreciation for certain types of property.

Under Section 179 of the Internal Revenue Code, taxpayers can elect to recover all or part of the cost of certain qualifying property, up to a limit, by deducting the cost of the property in the year the property is placed in service. This allows taxpayers to expense the property in the year placed in service, as opposed to taking depreciation deductions over a period of time.

To qualify for Section 179, property must be eligible property acquired, by purchase, for business use. Eligible property is tangible personal property, including off-the-shelf computer software. Tangible personal property is defined as any tangible property that is not real property. Off-the-shelf computer software is defined as software that is placed in service after 2002 and before 2006, readily available for purchase by the general public, subject to a nonexclusive license, and has not been substantially modified. It includes programs designed to cause a computer to perform a desired function. A database is not considered computer software unless it is in the public domain and is incidental to the operation of otherwise qualifying software.

The Section 179 deduction generally is the cost of the qualifying property up to a dollar amount established by law, currently $105,000. The amount of Section 179 deduction in any 1 year, however, cannot exceed the amount of business income. Furthermore, if the cost of the qualifying property placed in service during the year exceeds a dollar amount established by law, currently $420,000, the dollar limit must be reduced by the amount of cost over $420,000.

Special rules apply for depreciation and Section 179 deductions when dealing with listed property. Listed property includes cars, property used for entertainment, and certain computers and cellular phones.

Listed property must meet the business-use requirement. If the property is not used predominantly (more than 50%) for business, it must be depreciated using the straight-line method and is not eligible for Section 179 treatment.

Passenger automobiles have their own set of depreciation rules. Annual limits apply to depreciation deductions, including Section 179 deductions. A passenger automobile is considered any 4-wheeled vehicle made for use in public streets and rated at 6000 pounds or less of gross vehicle weight. The maximum amount of depreciation allowed for passenger automobiles as of the date of this publication is $3,060 for year 1; $4,900 for year 2; $2,950 for year 3; and $1,775 for year 4 and all years thereafter. These limits assume 100% business use and must be reduced by the percentage of personal use of the passenger automobile.

Passenger automobiles that have a gross vehicle weight exceeding 6000 pounds are not subject to the limits on depreciation for passenger automobiles but instead are treated as other 5-year assets for regular depreciation purposes. In regards to Section 179 deductions, vehicles weighing more that 6000 pounds qualify for up to $25,000 of Section 179 expense.

Tax laws and tax strategies

In 2004, four tax acts were passed by Congress and signed into law by the President. Some of the more relevant provisions, as they relate to physicians, are discussed herein.

Charitable deductions of vehicles

One change put into effect by the Jobs Creation Act of 2004 is in regard to the deductibility of vehicles when donated to charitable organizations. In the past, a taxpayer who donated a used automobile to a charitable donee generally deducted the fair market value, rather than the taxpayer's basis, when contributing the car. As a rule, a used car-pricing guide was used to determine the fair market value of the donated vehicle. Many times taxpayers realized a greater tax savings by donating the car than the cash they would receive if they sold the car outright. Under the new law, the charitable deduction is limited to subsequent sales proceeds. The deduction claim for vehicles, including automobiles, boats, and airplanes for which the claimed value exceeds $500 and excluding inventory property, depends on the use by the donee organization. If the donee organization sells the vehicle without any significant intervening use or material improvement of the vehicle, the amount of the deduction is limited to the gross proceeds received from the sale. The new law requires the charitable organization to issue a contemporaneous written acknowledgment that contains the name of the taxpayer, identification number of the taxpayer, vehicle identification number, and amount received for the vehicle sale. An acknowledgment is considered contemporaneous if it is provided within 30 days of the sale of the vehicle. If the charitable organization uses the vehicle in a manner connected with the organization, the donee must furnish an acknowledgment containing certification of the intended use or material improvement of the vehicle, intended duration of such use, and certification that the vehicle will not be transferred in exchange for money, other property, or services before completion of such use or improvement. The acknowledgment must be provided within 30 days of the contribution. A deduction is not allowed by the taxpayer unless such an acknowledgment is received.

Marriage relief penalty

Under EGRTTA '01, Congress addressed the marriage penalty in two ways. First, it increased the basic standard deduction for married individuals who file a joint return gradually to 200% of the amount allowed for single individual filers. This phase-in was scheduled to occur over a period of 5 years. In 2005, joint filers are allowed a standard deduction of 174% of single filers; in 2006 184%; in 2007 187%; in 2008 190%; and, in 2009 and after, 200% of the single filer. Second, it changed the break points for the tax rates to reflect twice the amount of income for the single filers. Under Jobs and Growth Tax Relief Reconciliation Act for 2003 (JGTRRA '03), for 2003 and 2004 only, the basic standard deduction for joint filers was accelerated to 200% of the amount for single filers. Under the Working Families Tax Relief Act of 2004, the provision has been expanded to include all tax years through 2010.

Capital gains rates

The new tax laws did not affect the lower capital gains rates enacted under JGTRRA '03. Long-term capital gains rates remain at 5% for lower income individuals and 15% for higher income individuals. These rates apply to tax years ending after May 5, 2003, and beginning before January 1, 2009. For 2008 only, the 5% rate is reduced to 0%. Tax rates for dividends from domestic corporations and qualified foreign corporations received by noncorporate taxpayers piggyback those rates. For purposes of determining long-term treatment for capital assets, the asset must be held for more than 1 year.

Health savings accounts

The Medicare Prescription Drug and Modernization Act of 2003 established health savings accounts (HSA). This is perhaps one of the most talked-about provisions enacted by any recent tax law. For tax years beginning after 2003, individuals or businesses may establish HSA. Into these HSA, tax-deductible contributions can be made under certain circumstances to pay qualified medical expenses of eligible individuals. Earnings on the HSA are tax-free and distributions from the HSA are tax-free to the extent they are used to pay for qualified medical expenses. Amounts contributed to an HSA that are not used in the current year roll over to successive tax years until distributed.

Eligible individuals who can contribute to HSA are defined as individuals who are (1) covered under a high deductible health plan, (2) not covered by any other health plan that is not a high deductible plan (with certain exceptions for plans that have limited and specific coverage), (3) not entitled to benefits under Medicare, and (4) not claimed as a dependent on another person's tax return.

High deductible health plans are defined as health plans that, for self-only coverage, have an annual deductible of at least $1000 and annual out-of-pocket expenses required to be paid (deductibles, copayments, and other amounts, but not premiums) not exceeding $5000. For family coverage, health plans must have an annual deductible of at least $2000 and annual out-of-pocket expenses not exceeding $10,000. In the case of in-network plans, these limits are applied using the in-network deductibles and copayments. In the case of family coverage, plans are a high deductible health plan only if, under the terms of the plan, no amounts are payable from the health plans until families incur annual covered medical expenses in excess of the minimum annual deductible. There is, however, an exception to this rule if the plans do not have a deductible or have a small deductible for preventive care coverage only. Preventive care is defined to include periodic health evaluations, such as annual physicals, routine prenatal and well-child care, child and adult immunizations, tobacco cessation and weight-loss programs, and screening services.

Certain exceptions are allowed to the provision that eligible individuals may not be covered under any health plan that is not a high deductible plan. Permitted insurances and permitted coverages do exist under the law. Permitted insurance is considered coverage under which substantially all of the coverage provided relates to liabilities incurred under workers' compensation laws, tort liabilities, liabilities relating to ownership or use of property, insurance for a specified disease or illness, and hospitalization insurance that pays a fixed amount per day or per other period. Permitted coverage, either through insurance or otherwise, is coverage for accidents, disability, dental care, vision care, or long-term care.

HSA can be established with a qualified HSA trustee or custodian with or without involvement by an employer. Qualified HSA trustees or custodians include any insurance company, bank, or any other person approved by the Internal Revenue Service (IRS) to be a trustee or custodian of individual retirement accounts or Archer medical savings accounts.

Employers and individuals can establish HSA. Employers, employees, or individuals may make HSA contributions. Employer contributions to HSA on employees' behalf are treated as employer-provided coverage for medical expenses under an accident or health plan and are excludable from the employees' gross income. Employer contributions are not subject to withholding from wages for income tax and are not subject to employment taxes. Contributions to employees' HSA through a cafeteria plan are treated as employer contributions. Contributions made by individuals to HSA are deductible by individuals as an adjustment to gross income on their returns.

Individuals can receive distributions from HSA at any time. Distributions used exclusively to pay for qualified medical expenses of individuals, their spouses, or dependents are excluded from gross income. Distributions that are not used for qualified medical expenses are includible in gross income and subject to an additional 10% tax. The penalty applies except in the cases of death, disability, or if the taxpayer turns 65. Qualified medical expenses are medical care expenses as defined by the IRS, including some nonprescription drugs. Distributions are not taxed if they are rolled over into another HSA within 60 days.

Health insurance premiums are not qualified medical expenses unless they are for qualified long-term care insurance, COBRA health care continuation coverage, or health care coverage while an individual is receiving unemployment compensation. Also, for individuals over age 65, premiums for Medicare Part A or B, Medicare health maintenance organizations, and the employees' share of premiums for employer-sponsored health insurance, including premiums for employer-sponsored retiree health insurance, can be paid from HSA. Premiums for Medigap policies are not qualified medical expenses.

HSA contributions must be made in cash and may not exceed the lesser of 100% of the annual deductible under the high deductible health plan or the maximum annual deductible as adjusted for inflation. Although these limits are expressed on an annual basis, they are calculated on a monthly basis. This allows individuals to participate in HSA in the first month they are eligible to do so. Additional HSA catch-up contributions are permitted for individuals or employees who are age 55 or older. The catch-up contribution amount is $600 in 2005, increasing in increments of $100 per year until 2009. Once employees reach age 65, no further contributions are permitted. Annual contributions made in excess of the allowed amounts are subject to a 6% excise tax until they are either distributed or applied to the HSA funding limit in a subsequent year. Contributions can be made any time during the tax year and at any time before the due date (without extensions) for the filing of the eligible individuals' income tax returns.

Upon the death of HSA account holders, a remaining account balance becomes the property of a named beneficiary. The account balance is included in the account holder's gross estate unless the account holder's surviving spouse is the named beneficiary, in which case the account becomes the property of the surviving spouse and the value of the account qualifies for the marital deductions. When beneficiaries are not an account holder's spouse, accounts ceases to be HSA and beneficiaries must include the date-of-death balance in current income. The amount included in income may be reduced by any amounts that are expended from HSA within 1 year after the death of decedents to pay qualified medical expenses of decedents. HSA transfers made in connection with a divorce are not taxable and the transferred assets are treated thereafter as HSA.

Given the fact that HSA are in their infancy, there are many administrative details that have not yet been addressed and information continues to be forthcoming.

Other tax considerations

Tax planning for divorce

Tax planning for life-changing events sometimes is an area that is overlooked, especially in the area of divorce. The following is a list of the top 10 mistakes made in divorce situations:

- Splitting assets between husband and wife without considering the property's basis
- Losing the benefit of the child tax credit, HOPE, and lifetime learning credit
- Assuming that the payment of attorney and expert fees are deductible

- Not analyzing the best filing status for the tax return
- Disguising child support as alimony
- Not specifying that alimony ends at death
- Assuming that the capital gains tax is based on client's share of the proceeds
- Letting alimony payments drop off too quickly
- Fighting over the dependency exemption when one party cannot use it
- Not consulting a tax expert

Although tax considerations should not be a major factor when making life-changing decisions, they should be considered to minimize unpleasant surprises.

Alternative minimum tax planning

The alternative minimum tax (AMT) plays a major role in tax planning. AMT applies if it exceeds the amount calculated under the regular tax method. AMT is computed by applying a 26% rate on the first $175,000 of alternative minimum taxable income (AMTI) and 28% on the amount of AMTI in excess of $175,000. The AMT rate for AMTI between $150,000 and $330,000 may be as high as 30%. If AMT applies, certain deductions may not provide tax benefits, because they may have to be added back either as an AMT adjustment or an AMT tax preference item. The amount deducted for regular tax purposes for personal exemptions also is required to be added back in computing AMTI. Some of the more common add-backs for AMT purposes include medical and dental expenses; taxes from Schedule A; certain interest on a home mortgage not used to buy, build, or improve a principal residence; miscellaneous deductions; and exercise of incentive stock options.

AMT makes it more difficult to assess individual tax situations. For example, under the regular tax system, individuals who pay their fourth-quarter state tax estimate in the current tax year receive a tax benefit for doing so. Prepaying the fourth-quarter estimate, however, because it is an add-back for AMT purposes, may result in AMT and, therefore, no benefit is realized for regular tax purposes. The number of taxpayers caught in the AMT net has increased significantly in the past several years. Careful consideration should be given to AMT planning to attempt to minimize the burden it imposes.

Retirement plan strategies

Retirement plans are one of the few great tax benefits available to physicians. Many retirement plan options are available to physicians (discussed elsewhere in this issue) Suffice to say, physicians, when reviewing their retirement plan options, should involve plan experts to help them make the best possible decisions.

Summary

Accountants are not mind readers. More importantly, it is difficult and sometimes impossible to change bad business outcomes or bad tax consequences after the fact. Involve accountants proactively and get advice, especially on major business decisions.

The medical profession is one in which there are changes in every area of practice on an ongoing basis. The profession is inundated with changes in technology, new and better techniques, medications, and so forth. In addition to the medical side of the equation, regulations make it more and more difficult to operate a practice. The alphabet soup of OSHA, CLIA, HIPAA, and other laws, such as Stark, that relate specifically to the medical profession are overwhelming, at best. Throw into the mix the everyday stress of running a business, personnel issues, tax issues, capitalization issues, and so forth, and physicians have more than a full-time job. Having competent accountants who can assist physicians in managing their practices and making the right decisions is crucial.

ELSEVIER
SAUNDERS

Urol Clin N Am 32 (2005) 271–273

UROLOGIC
CLINICS
of North America

Negotiating Insurance Contracts—Is There Any Hope?

Cindy Spears

Dean, Dorton & Ford, PSC, 106 West Vine Street, Suite 600, Lexington, KY 40507, USA

During most of the twentieth century, physicians were in charge of their own reimbursements for services they provided. During this period, before the 1980s, there were few mandates or regulations regarding the services they provided; there were no bundling issues, no modifiers, and no written referrals. Physicians and their staff focused on healing patients, not on a business plan. The end of the century, however, brought new challenges and a completely different environment for health care providers. One of these changes is the responsibility of physicians to negotiate insurance contracts. Although this is a difficult task, the good news is that it can be done. This article outlines the ways to negotiate an insurance contract successfully.

Where do these changes leave physicians and their practices?

Physicians were left with decreases in reimbursement that often did not cover the costs of providing services. Physicians had to make choices as to which commercial insurance companies they could afford to participate with. Practices also had to jump through hoops to get claims paid while lowering overhead to be profitable. Physicians began to question if they had to accept the proposed reimbursement or the current reimbursement and decide if they could negotiate for better rates. These negotiations have proven effective and generate better reimbursement for physicians. It is difficult to have the same result or success in negotiating with various payers and it is dependent on the state. There are, however, guidelines to follow when attempting to negotiate.

Where to begin?

The process begins with gathering information about the market and then determining the importance of a practice's presence in the marketplace. It is more difficult to negotiate in a market that is saturated with a practice specialty versus a market that needs a specialty. The market typically is considered a geographic area, but, in this instance, the market is defined by a physician panel for the insurance company and the number of physicians in the specialty in the entire geographic region. If insurance companies are marketing to a large company or moving into new geographic territories, they want to be able to market a large base of providers of all specialties. In this instance, providers have more leverage and the payers are more receptive to negotiations.

To determine the specialty presence in the market, go to internet sites for the various payers and look up participating providers. Although these lists generally are not completely accurate, they are a starting point. It is advisable to call the physicians on the list and verify their participation with an insurance company.

After the amount of leverage is determined, then what?

Once leverage is determined and the decision is made to negotiate with a payer, it is time to gather the data necessary to support an increase in reimbursement and make an action plan for negotiations. One question to ask at this point is, "Can someone in the practice conduct the negotiations or is it necessary to hire an outside consultant to coordinate the process?" There are three basic strategies a practice can follow in contract negotiations.

0094-0143/05/$ - see front matter © 2005 Elsevier Inc. All rights reserved.
doi:10.1016/j.ucl.2005.03.007

urologic.theclinics.com

What are the strategies and how to know which is best for a practice?

The first strategy is for a practice to complete negotiations without using outside resources. The second is to hire a consultant to perform the negotiation. The third is for a practice to join a physician network. This type of network was developed to help physicians gain bargaining power. The network negotiates as a group versus each practice negotiating for itself. This strategy has proven beneficial in certain regions with certain payers but is not a sure shot to better negotiations. The first two strategies, a practice performing its own negotiations and a practice hiring a consultant, are similar in approach, each having strengths and weaknesses.

The strengths for practices completing the negotiations themselves are cost and control. It can be costly to hire someone to negotiate a contract and sometimes the end result of the negotiation is not substantial. Also, practices keep more control if they do not hire someone else to perform negotiations. The main weakness with keeping negotiations internal is that many times managers or physicians do not have the time to dedicate to the process or they lack the extensive experience necessary to conduct a successful negotiation.

The strengths for hiring consultants are experience and expertise. Consultants often have developed rapport with the payers, and they have knowledge of reimbursement trends in the market. Also, working regularly with payers creates a familiarity with the process, providing much-needed expertise. Be aware that although developing relationships with payers typically is a strength, it also can be a weakness. If consultants have allegiances to particular payers, those relationships can hinder them from advocating aggressively for practices.

To determine which strategy to use, practices should inquire as to which method has worked best in the market. Some geographic areas have strong physician networks, whereas others have none. If there are no physician networks or a practice chooses to go another route, then consultants should be interviewed to determine their ability and experience in negotiating physician contracts. It often works best to have consultants perform the analysis and be go-betweens between practices and the payers, while keeping practices actively involved and notified of each step. Consultants always should be advocating for practices' best interests. Regardless of the strategy, there

are steps to follow in gathering the data and preparing the analysis.

After determining a negotiations strategy, what information should be gathered?

- Determine reimbursement by CPT code for the payer.
- Run a frequency report for the payer (a report for the most recent 12-month period that includes CPT code, frequency of CPT code, and the dollar amount charged and reimbursed for the code).
- Determine method of current reimbursement currently (RVUs, percent of Medicare, and so forth).
- Determine the proposed reimbursement amount and the means to determine (150% of Medicare, $65 conversion factor); make this amount higher than expected to allow room for negotiation.
- Determine the minimal amount of increase that will be accepted and the consequences if the demands are not met (eg, terminate contract).
- Determine how the payer reimburses for items pertinent to the practice, such as:
  - Midlevel providers
  - Injections
  - Laboratory work in the office
  - Procedures specific to the specialty
  - Modifiers
  - Payment for multiple procedures
- Review old explanation of benefits (EOB) to see if there are issues with reimbursement accuracy, rejections, or length of time to receive the payment.
- Review current contract for issues that need to be addressed (eg, filing limit).
- Determine procedures or services where reimbursement does not cover the cost to perform services.
- Make a list of negotiation topics (eg, inflators: rate increases each year over a period of time).

Once the information is analyzed and in place, contact the insurance company representative to schedule a meeting. It is important to have all bases covered and strong support for reimbursement demands. It also is important to review issues other than reimbursement during this meeting. For example, address problems related to billing, such as delayed payments, filing limit not allowing enough time, and modifiers not recognized.

What is needed to prepare for a meeting with an insurance payer?

In preparation for a meeting with a payer representative, prepare a simple document that includes current reimbursement rates, proposed reimbursement rates, and other negotiation topics. This initial meeting serves as a means to provide a proposal to the payer. Most likely there is no actual negotiating at this meeting. The negotiation process can be lengthy and may encompass several meetings. Because of this lengthy process, it is important to establish a timeline for payers that clearly states the expectations of practices.

Another topic of discussion at an initial meeting is which process the insurance company uses to determine increases in rates now and in the future. If a carrier bases reimbursement on RVUs or the Medicare fee schedule, it is important to know which year it uses and how often it is updated. Also, ask the representative for any reports that may be beneficial (eg, payment data from their system on certain codes).

What happens next?

Most likely, insurance company representatives take proposals and conduct reviews and analyses themselves with their data, then come back with a counterproposal. Once a practice receives the counterproposal, it should look for areas of acceptance and areas it is not willing to accept. This narrows down the issues to stand firm on. The practice then should develop a counterproposal and provide any additional supporting documentation. The practice may have EOBs from other payers showing another carrier pays more for certain codes, which can be supplied to support the requested increase. Also, if there are invoices for supplies indicating that the costs to perform a procedure are more than what is reimbursed, the invoices can be supplied for support. There may be several counterproposals throughout the process. The practice has to decide how firm it is going to be and what is non-negotiable. Throughout the proposal and counter-proposals, spreadsheets should be kept as to the expected dollar increases by using frequency reports. These spreadsheets should show the actual cumulative expected dollar increases, which can be used to assess the need to continue in negotiations.

What happens if an agreement cannot be reached?

If an agreement cannot be reached, then a practice must decide if it terminates the contract or agrees to accept what is offered. If the terms are agreed to, then the contract is signed with an effective date. The contract should be reviewed closely to ensure all terms are accurate and stated clearly. Payments received after the effective date should be reviewed for accuracy and audits should be performed periodically to ensure there are no changes made to reimbursement.

Once the contract is signed, how does a practice know the negotiations are a success?

Look at the bottom line. Is the expected revenue amount substantial enough to support a practice participating with a payer, and does it pay for the time and resources it took to negotiate?

Payers still have the majority of the control over reimbursement; however, physicians can negotiate terms effectively and achieve reimbursements with a positive outcome. These may be baby steps, but they are steps forward. Now, if there only were hope for malpractice rates.

ELSEVIER
SAUNDERS

Urol Clin N Am 32 (2005) 275–284

UROLOGIC
CLINICS
of North America

Medical Records Management—Steps Toward a Paperless Environment

Rick Rutherford, CMPE

American Urological Association, 1000 Corporate Boulevard, Linthicum, MD 21090, USA

Like many surgical specialists, urologists in private practice are faced with a quandary about the least expensive, but most effective, method of managing the flow of medical records in their patient care activities. Pressures continue to build from various forces toward a rapid and seamless exchange of patient health information between myriad health care stakeholders. Entities that pay for health care demand more and more data to justify shrinking reimbursements. The spiraling litigiousness of a more educated, more demanding society increases the need for accurate and thorough documentation of health care procedures. Enhanced patient mobility demands that individual private health information must follow patients anywhere in the world. All these forces drive practitioners toward improvements in handling their patients' medical records, but no help is in sight to offset the expenses associated with a conversion from a record-keeping process that evolved in a closed system to one that allows interchanges between health care providers, not just in the local provider community but anywhere patients may find themselves in need of health care.

Historical perspective

Since the early days of the medical profession, the necessity for careful record keeping has been a cornerstone of the art. The continuum of medical care dictates that physicians must record carefully the diagnostic findings and interventional steps taken to ensure that future treatment incorporates a consistent and progressive approach to the

solution of health care problems. The origins of safeguarding personal medical information are found in the Hippocratic oath: "What I may see or hear in the course of the treatment or even outside of the treatment in regard to the life of men, which on no account one must spread abroad, I will keep to myself, holding such things shameful to be spoken about" [1]. In the early days, notes on patient care were kept in physicians' own handwriting and considered the property of physicians, to be shared with no one, not even patients. The specialization of medicine and the democratic process in the United States have led to a health care environment in which information concerning patients' care must be divulged to many other health care providers and their employees to provide the quality of care that they have come to expect. Only with the passage of the Health Insurance Portability and Accountability Act of 1996 (HIPAA) have the methods of sharing health care information and the access rights of providers and patients been codified.

A typical records management model

Medical records management in today's typical urology practices still is based on a paper process. Each health care entity's physicians and employees maintain the basic patient medical records, the charts, in a closed system. Urologists see patients, dictate (or in some cases handwrite) the findings, which then are added to the charts. Information from these records to be transmitted to other specialists or back to patients' primary care physicians is sent in print format by mail or fax. When physicians or members of a staff need to reference this information, original charts must be located

E-mail address: rrutherford@auanet.org

0094-0143/05/$ - see front matter © 2005 Elsevier Inc. All rights reserved.
doi:10.1016/j.ucl.2005.03.009

urologic.theclinics.com

and transported to the locations where reviews are conducted. With the advent of multiple sites for the delivery of care, the process of locating charts and delivering them has become expensive and problematic. The processing of information has led to the creation of a specialized occupation, the medical records and health information technician [2]. In 2002, approximately 147,000 people were employed as medical records and health information technicians in the United States [2], 63% of whom were employed in nonhospital settings. Several professional organizations offer certification credentials in the medical records field, such as the registered health information technician certified by the American Health Information Management Association. To qualify for registered health information technician certification, health information technicians must have an associate's degree from an accredited program and must pass a written examination. According to the 2002 United States Department of Labor survey data, the average salary for health information technicians in a physician's office is $21,320 [2].

The primary purpose for patient charts is to assure continuity of care. In addition to records of urologists' encounters with individual patients, charts contain records of laboratory tests, radiographic studies, hospital care, and copies of records from other physicians involved in patients' care. Record technicians have developed processes to help organize the information to assist the health care provider in efficient review of historical data while assessing patients' current condition. Charts are subdivided into sections for laboratory records, correspondence from other caregivers, and so forth. Within these subdivisions, records are filed chronologically, so that physicians can browse through the information to pick out facts and figures pertinent to a patient's current problem. With paper charts, it is difficult, if not impossible, for urologists to access immediately individual data items without paging through several documents. This is time consuming and mentally taxing. More time can be wasted in simply locating particular patients' charts in order to respond to phone calls than it takes to carry on the phone conversation. Because several employees of a urology team may need the data contained in individual charts at any given time, the chart location not always is determined easily. Consider an example of a patient scheduled for an inpatient procedure: the scheduling secretary needs the chart to precertify the procedure with the patient's insurance company; the nurse needs it to schedule preoperative testing; another staff member needs it to send copies of the most recent note to the primary care doctor; and the physician may have incomplete dictation to finish before the surgery. In the most efficient system, all of these tasks may be completed simultaneously, but because there is only one paper chart per patient, it must be passed from individual to individual, slowing down the work process for everyone. In the past decade or so, this inefficiency has been the driving force in the trend toward electronic data recording and storage. If the chart is virtual, every need for information can be satisfied simultaneously.

Progress toward electronic health records

Despite the efficiencies to be gained in moving toward a paperless medical records management system, average urologists are hesitant to make the leap toward electronic health records (EHR). A recent survey reports that only 15% of primary care physicians currently use EHR [3]. The percentage of users is even lower among urologists. Nationally, only approximately 1 in 10 urologists currently use electronic medical record keeping in their practice setting [4]. Certain regions of the country are involved more heavily. Nearly 25% of urologists responding to a survey conducted by the Western Section of the American Urological Association report using electronic medical records [5]. Although several physicians in each survey indicate their intent to adopt EHR in the near future, there clearly are significant barriers that must be overcome to sway the majority of practicing urologists to step into the virtual record-keeping world (discussed later).

Physicians who are using EHR as their primary means of medical records management are fairly consistent in which tasks are completed electronically. The majority of users document their patient encounters electronically either by inserting transcribed dictation or using electronic templates that allow physicians to chart by exception. Many systems allow physicians to use e-prescribing to transmit patient prescriptions to pharmacies. Most software allows transfer of demographic data from practice management systems to the electronic medical records to save keystrokes. Many users harness the power of EHR to assist in generating charges for patient services [3].

Voice recognition software has yet to become a prevalent method of dictating for physicians using EHR. The inefficiency associated with training even the most sophisticated voice recognition systems prevents busy practitioners from mastering its use. Many EHR users rely on customized word-processing templates to improve the speed with which they can generate patient notes to be stored in their systems. Vendors have stimulated this behavior by sharing templates designed by specialists with customers who then modify the notes to fit their own practice style. Other templates are built into notepad-sized computers using checkboxes that physicians mark with an electronic stylus to indicate which examination steps have been completed. Each checkbox drives a standard phrase so that physicians build the note electronically as examinations are completed.

Return on investment remains unclear

The cost of acquiring and implementing electronic medical records is substantial. Most urologists faced with dwindling Medicare reimbursements for services find it difficult to justify investments with no clear return. The efficiencies gained often are intangible and have more to do with improving lifestyle for busy physicians than with improving revenue or reducing overhead costs. Larger group practices with existing economies of scale and centralized functions are more successful at demonstrating true cost reductions. During a recent Medical Group Management Association (MGMA) audioconference, the administrator of a pediatric center with 14 providers pointed out that the primary savings to their clinic from implementing EHR was attributable to reduced personnel costs. By reducing the number of paper charts pulled from 436,140 per year to 67,527 per year, the clinic was able to reduce clerical support staff by 10 full-time equivalents for an annual payroll savings of $160,000 [6]. In smaller practices, however, where the support staff often is responsible for clinical tasks and administrative tasks, it is more difficult to achieve a direct reduction in payroll costs by reducing administrative tasks, with the exception of reduced overtime. It is more likely that costs of electronic medical records hardware and software could be recovered through increased revenue. Areas of improvement that may be possible include more accurate coding with the help of the interactive checklists (discussed previously), reductions in missed charges, and reductions in denied claims based on better documentation. Another recent survey by the Medical Records Institute shows that 74.8% of physicians and nurses list "improved clinical documentation to support appropriate billing service levels" as a factor driving the need for EHR systems [7]. Still, no clear-cut evidence exists that demonstrates a positive cash flow based on the implementation of EHR. Conventional wisdom supports the fact that some form of government funding is necessary to encourage urologists in small groups to take the plunge. The same survey shows that more than 55% of respondents list "lack of adequate funding or resources" as the chief barrier to implementation [7].

Application options for electronic health records

In the current environment, medical groups may choose to adopt electronic record-keeping processes in one of several ways. The choice often is driven by the capital equipment and annual maintenance costs of the solutions considered, counterbalanced with practices' desire to move toward a completely paperless environment.

Some smaller practices, facing a dwindling amount of space to store paper records, opt for the use of a document imaging management system (DIMS). All patient information is recorded on paper, but the documents generated by practices and those received from outside are scanned into digital format and stored in a database that allows search and access by multiple users. This helps eliminate the inefficiency of having only a single access to patient information, reduces the problem of missing charts, and drastically reduces the storage space needed for paper charts. A DIMS does not, however, assist in improved billing documentation, does nothing to facilitate support of clinical decision making, and contributes only slightly to improved quality of care. Many more sophisticated electronic medical records packages use DIMS technology to store and manage nondigital documentation from outside sources or to provide a rapid conversion pathway to link old patient charts to new electronic health information recorded after EHR implementation. The future of DIMS is not clear in light of the United States government's push toward complete interoperability of patient health records by the year 2014 [8].

For urology practices that choose to acquire software designed to create a true electronic record, the range of options is enormous. Several hundred vendors currently market products in the United States and abroad that run on hardware ranging from stand-alone personal computers to mainframe systems. The majority of EHR users today operate their software on client servers that allow networking of personal computers and notebooks to a central data repository. Some of these even operate over the internet using what is described as application service provider software. This option is unique in that it can be purchased on a monthly licensing basis, which carries a lower price tag than proprietary systems. There are concerns among EHR shoppers about the security of the private health information data transmitted via the internet. The National Health Information Technical Coordinator, David Brailer, however, appointed recently by President Bush, mentioned a "medical internet controlled by the patient" as an option for the solution to the interoperability goal of the President's plan [9].

Potential for improvement in patient safety and quality

Brailer points out that there is evidence that implementation of EHR can improve the safety of health care delivery and improve the quality of services rendered. Brailer mentions more than 60 peer-reviewed articles that analyze the benefits to patients of electronic record keeping in terms of improved longevity and safety [9]. Clearly, the ability of all members of a health care team to have immediate access to current medical data about given patients serves to minimize the number of medical errors that occur in the United States. The factor driving the need for EHR mentioned most often in the Medical Records Institute survey of physicians and nurses is the need to improve the quality of care (87.4% of respondents mentioned that need). In addition, 73.1% of them list the need to reduce medical errors [7].

The Medicare Modernization Act of 2004 contains language requiring implementation of e-prescribing processes for any drug plans covered by the Medicare prescription drug benefit. An electronic prescription system could reduce errors attributable to illegible handwriting and assuage the problem of adverse drug interactions by reviewing new prescriptions against those already recorded on patients' EHR [10].

Access to patients' up-to-date health information is vital to providing the best possible care. It

is for that reason that the Joint Commission on Accreditation of Healthcare Organizations specifies standards for completion of medical records, and many hospitals have stringent disciplinary policies for noncompletion of patient records. According to Doyon, "the implementation of electronic medical records will improve the quality of the documentation within the record and may also reduce the number of deficiencies noted" [11].

Integration of performance measures into an EHR system not only can improve patient care but also reduce overall costs. The American Medical Association formed a Physician Consortium for Performance Improvement that adopted performance measures intended to enhance the quality of patient care. In a recent article in the *AMNews*, the Midwest Heart Specialists in greater Chicago report that after integrating some of the consortium performance measures on coronary artery disease into their EHR, their practice had fewer deaths, heart attacks, and strokes than similar patients in other published studies. In addition, hospitalization costs were reduced by more than $3 million [12].

Barriers to adoption of electronic health records

Despite the buzz about EHR and its benefits, the adoption rate has been slow to increase. The most frequently cited barrier to widespread adoption in every survey is related to cost. This is a legitimate concern. Health care provider spending on information technology in the United States in 2004 was nearly $16 billion [13]. According to Forrester Research, sales for electronic medical records to physician practices will climb from $816 million in 2003 to $1.4 billion in 2008. Small physician practices, which make up less than half the sales, are expected to increase to 60% of total sales by 2008 [14]. Although competition is driving the EHR price per user down, the cost of hardware and software to install a system averages from $15,000 to $30,000 per physician [15]. Other barriers cited include the following:

- Lack of support by the medical staff
- Difficulty in finding a turnkey solution from one vendor
- Difficulty in planning the conversion from paper to EHR
- Lack of standardization of code sets and terminologies

- Difficulty in evaluating choices with no set standards [16]

In a recent speech at the MGMA 2004 Annual Conference, Brailer explained that approximately half of EHR implementation projects fail [17]. This statistic combined with the lack of available capital to invest in a system creates the impression of immense risk in making the right choice. Physicians naturally are skeptical of new and unproven techniques, and when they are asked to sink their own economic resources into an investment of this magnitude, the lack of enthusiasm is not surprising. Add to that the concern that implementing EHR requires significant changes in their routines for the gathering and use of medical information in day-to-day patient care, and the hesitancy to adopt EHR among urologists in small groups is almost insurmountable. Many forces are at play to stimulate greater interest in widespread conversion to EHR, but the momentum toward change is not there yet.

Electronic health records product selection process

In typical urology practices, the responsibility for evaluating various medical record packages falls to a practice administrator and one or more physicians who have declared an interest in making the change. Most experts declare that without a visionary physician-champion to lobby for change among the other stakeholders, the switch to a paperless record-keeping system is impossible. In a recent MGMA article, Halich, co-chair of the MGMA Information Technology Advisory Panel, states, "Support from physicians is by far the most important critical success factor..." [17]. Selection of appropriate software is a daunting and time-consuming process, because there are few recognized data sources that include all available choices of software for practices of every size. The lack of consumer-oriented information restricts approaching the selection of an EHR product in a scientific method. The Medical Records Institute sponsors an annual meeting of the Toward Electronic Patient Records Conference and Exhibition, where awards are presented to the highest-rated software packages as reviewed by volunteers. KLAS Enterprises produces a series of reports based on satisfaction survey responses from health care information technology executives, department directors, and managers [18]. This is the nearest type of *Consumer Reports*–style publication that

exists in the industry, but one criticism of the KLAS reports is that they lack direct input from physician end-users. Currently, no certification process exists that allows EHR software vendors to demonstrate that the product they market meets generally accepted specifications. The selection team must gather information from a variety of sources and hope that some of the packages that seem appropriate actually turn out to be a fit for their practice. Many practices hire a consultant to guide them in determining which features will prove most valuable to the physicians in a practice and how to prepare for the conversion with a minimum of headaches.

The evaluation process normally includes issuing requests for proposals (RFP) to potential vendors by a urology practice. The RFP allows the gathering of specific critical information from each vendor to be considered in the selection process. The request should provide information about the practice, the perceived needs for electronic information, descriptions of existing hardware and software, expectations about the information-passing capability between the new software and the old system and clear guidance about what the parameters of an acceptable proposal are. The vendor's response to an RFP reflects the cost projections for implementation and for annual hardware and software maintenance, the proposed implementation timeline, and a specimen purchase contract. It also should contain financial information about the company, specifications about database management, integration features, the potential for interoperability with other medical information systems, and references [19]. Based on responses to these requests, the products to be considered are scheduled for a demonstration in front of a group of key decision makers for the practice, referred to as the product selection team (PST). This team normally consists of a practice administrator, physicians who lead the practice's providers in the usage, and staff members who regularly make use of the existing practice records. The demonstration should be based on specific scenarios provided by the practice, using actual patient demographic and clinical information that has been altered to protect the confidentiality of the patients. This mock patient database and the series of challenge scenarios should be designed by the PST and be presented consistently to each vendor in advance of the demonstration date. As the demonstration is conducted, features should be rated using a consistent scale and any questions posed by the PST should be recorded carefully along with the answers. Any answers to be provided later by the vendor should have a deadline established before the conclusion of the product demonstration. After the demonstration, representatives of the PST should contact other urology practices that currently use the product and someone from the PST should make a site visit to see how the software operates in a live environment compared with a demonstration environment. It is prudent to try to identify active users of the product beyond those given on a vendor's reference list. Such information can be solicited through internet forums, listservs, and professional associations. After all demonstrations are completed, the number of choices is narrowed to two or three that are deemed satisfactory and negotiation of price, with included features, takes place. It is good business practice to select two suitable vendors and software packages, because that allows stronger negotiation positions on price and service after purchase. The entire selection process from issuance of the RFP to a go-live date (the actual day on which the software is installed and ready to use for real patients) often takes 6 months to 1 year.

Compliance issues associated with electronic health records

For urologists, compliance with the ever-increasing number of federal and state regulations connected with the management of patients' medical information has become a way of life. Government-funded programs to pay for health care services make up more than half of average urologists' annual revenue [20]. With this much of the reimbursement pie at stake, practices must consider carefully the ramifications that selection and implementation of EHR will have on their sundry compliance programs.

Fraud and abuse compliance

Medicare compliance and avoidance of fraud and abuse place tremendous emphasis on adequate documentation of services in the Medicare beneficiaries' medical records. The use of EHR must enhance the ability of urologists to construct an accurate summary of services rendered to patients to assure that payments received are not called into question. Computerization of information processes can save time and money through electronic shortcuts, but a practice compliance officer must be sure that the shortcuts do not undermine the accuracy of information reported to the government. In the modern era of EHR, physicians can expect that a template-generated note can justify more confidence in the level of coding payable for a particular patient encounter. If a system has design flaws that lead to overbilling or false claims being filed, however, then the savings are miniscule compared with the increased risk of fines. The implementation of EHR does not relieve urologists of the need for chart auditing to assure compliance with the latest Medicare coding and billing guidelines. It may improve the efficiency of the process, allowing for more thorough reviews. Nevertheless, installation of EHR signals the need for more auditing, retraining, and corrections in the short term rather than less.

Health Insurance Portability and Accountability Act of 1996 compliance

The compliance guidance associated with HIPAA "evolved and was passed, in part, to improve the efficiency and effectiveness of the health care system by standardizing the transmission of certain administrative and financial information and by protecting the privacy and security of personal health information" [21]. The electronic maintenance, storage, and transmission of confidential health information are precisely the activities that HIPAA is designed to control. Three important HIPAA rules have and will continue to have critical effects on the use of electronic health care information. These are the privacy rule, the security rule, and the electronic transaction and code sets rule. The privacy rule controls what personal health information must be safeguarded, how access can be granted or denied, and who is authorized to access the information in addition to patients and physicians who create it. When urology practices elect to implement EHR, the privacy of the data to be entered into the system must be a key point of concern. For example, employees of vendors who assist in converting existing information into EHR must be governed by a Business Associate Agreement, specified by HIPAA, to ensure that the information they handle remains confidential. The security rules deal with the processes used to create, store, and transmit electronic health data. Part of the outcry for standardization and certification of EHR packages comes from the need for users to guarantee that they are employing proper security measures to prevent unauthorized disclosures of confidential information. This means that anyone who accesses the electronic medical record must follow specific password protocols and safeguard computer terminals so that persons who have no need for access do not see what information is on the display. By the same token, in truly paperless environments, what assurance do patients and doctors have that the information vital to successful treatment will be there the next time it is needed? The security rule requires that users address backup procedures and redundancy to avoid lost data. The transaction and code set rules provide a road map to the interoperability, which is the key to allowing patient information to follow patients to any health care setting. The ability to transmit data from one site to another is useful only if senders and receivers can review and add to patients' health records. Without standardized data sets and electronic language specifications, the expansion of EHR will result in a health care tower of Babel with similar disastrous results.

Professional and governmental efforts to foster adoption

With an executive order issued by President Bush in April 2004 and the subsequent appointment of a czar of health care information technology, the handwriting clearly is on the wall about the future of EHR. The road to universal usage is not going to be as easy, however, as it will be in Canada and the United Kingdom, two countries also in the early stages of movements to widespread EHR use. Although the United States government has tremendous sway over health care because of the dollars under its control, it does not own the health care system, as is the case in the other two countries. In the United States, the Department of Health and Human Services (HHS) controls approximately 50% of the total health care dollars earned by urologists, whereas in the United Kingdom, the National Health System controls 85% of health care delivery and employs virtually all the urologists [22]. What forces will push the interest in EHR to the tipping point? They may be a combination of the following:

- Physician's Electronic Health Record Coalition (PEHRC)—an assemblage of the major primary-care and specialty societies committed to taking practical steps to educate physicians in small and medium-sized prac-

tices about the value and best use of EHR, to assist doctors in selection of systems, and to help focus the market on high-quality and affordable products. PEHRC represents more than 500,000 United States physicians. Additionally, PEHRC will work to participate in the development of the EHR certification process. Members of PEHRC currently serve in several workgroups connected with the design of a process to certify EHR software and to establish minimum functionality standards. In addition, PEHRC is assisting the MGMA Center for Research to conduct an information technology assessment on current usage patterns of EHR.
- Certification Commission for Health Information Technology (CCHIT)—a group of information technology experts formed to develop a process to certify health care information technology products [23]. By adopting certification standards, CCHIT can assist in boosting the confidence of health care providers that EHR investment is worth the risk. In addition, a certifying body will encourage vendors to target their research and development toward an interoperable environment based on the networking of local and national health information users. CCHIT is made up of four task forces with specific tasks designed to flesh out the certification process. These task forces are concerned with functionality, interoperability, security, and the actual certification and testing process.
- E-Health Initiative—the objective of this organization is to focus information technology efforts on the improvement of patient safety and the quality of health care services and improve the value of EHR [23]. The workgroup will suggest standard business practices and model contracts to support the acquisition process. It also will participate in discussions of standards that facilitate rapid data exchange among EHR and other clinical information systems.
- Doctors' Office Quality–Information Technology—a demonstration project supported by funds from the Centers for Medicare and Medicaid Services to improve the quality of care for Medicare beneficiaries through usage of EHR [23]. The 2-year demonstration project will test an integrated approach to specific disease management processes using EHR and the ability to transmit information electronically among participating providers.

- Health Level Seven Functional Standard (HL7)—the task of developing standards for the use and exchange of health care information falls to a list of standards setting organizations, such as HL7. They propose a set of functions essential to EHR. The functions will be used and tested by health care providers over a 2-year period and then the revised standards and the testing results submitted to the American National Standards Institute for approval as the approved standard that will determine how EHR packages will work in the future [23].
- Workgroup for Electronic Data Interchange—this advisory group has existed for more than 10 years. It provides advice to the government through the Secretary of HHS on a variety of health care information issues, such as HIPAA privacy, security, and national identifiers. Recently, it has developed working groups on EHR and e-prescribing.
- Council on the Application of Health Information Technology (CAHIT)—the federal government not only is an overseer and payer of health care services but also a provider of services. In this respect, the usage of EHR by government agencies, such as HHS and Veterans Administration (VA), are coordinated by CAHIT. Activities include development of a version of the VA's Veterans Health Information Systems and Technology Architecture Office EHR for use by non-VA physician offices. The first release of this product is expected in 2005 [24].

Vision of the paperless urology office

Urologists historically have made great strides in technologic development. From the prostatic blind punch to microwave thermotherapy, technologic advancement has driven immense improvements in patient care. These improvements required urologists to master new and radically different techniques regularly; the move toward electronic record keeping is no less demanding and, hopefully, no less rewarding. Urology's early adopters tout the amount of time saved in creating and maintaining records, once the processes become second nature to them. The real untapped benefit that will come with widespread adoption and the interconnectivity that will accompany it will be better patient care of genitourinary problems and better outcomes through information sharing.

Imagine a urology office in 2020. Mr. Jones is 56 years old and experiences difficulty in urination as he prepares for work one morning. During his first break at work, he accesses his personal genome profile that shows his current risk of benign prostatic hyperplasia and prostate cancer. He accesses the website, www.UrologyHealth.org [25], does some research on urinary problems, and then performs a search for urologists in his area. After selecting a board-certified urologist in his community, Dr. Brown, he links to the doctor's website where he browses the available new patient appointments and selects a slot that is convenient for his work schedule. He records his initial symptoms and enters his contact information. His appointment with Dr. Brown is confirmed for 1 week from Thursday. Arriving at home that night, he opens an e-mail message from the urologist's office, which welcomes him as a new patient and asks him to go to a secure link on Dr. Brown's web page, where he authorizes access to his electronic medical record stored in the regional health record repository. When he submits the authorization code, the system automatically downloads his complete medical history and billing information to Dr. Brown's computer system and instantly issues an e-mail message to Mr. Jones's primary care physician, alerting her to his upcoming appointment with the urologist. Dr. Brown's electronic medical record system has a built-in, clinical decision-making module that prepares a standard set of laboratory tests to be ordered for Mr. Jones. After dinner that night, Dr. Brown checks his e-mail inbox and reviews and approves the laboratory orders. This generates an encrypted e-mail message to Mr. Jones with a link to the laboratory, where he selects a convenient time to have the appropriate specimens collected and authorizes access to his information. His confirmation e-mail message provides him with instructions as to what to expect at the laboratory and indicates that the results will be sent automatically to Dr. Brown and downloaded into Mr. Jones's permanent electronic record.

On the day of his appointment, Mr. Jones arrives and is shown to a private computer kiosk where he reviews the information on file in his record, makes any corrections, and enters his personal password to verify authenticity. The computer system's web camera takes a snapshot and stores it in the EHR so that Dr. Brown's nurse can identify Mr. Jones in the reception area and escort him back to the examination area without mentioning his name in front of other patients.

Dr. Brown, while having his morning coffee, has reviewed and responded to all his morning e-mail messages from his nurse and patients. He has reviewed Mr. Jones's chart and his recent laboratory work. Using an electronic stylus, he indicates in a series of checkboxes which components of an examination he intends to perform, based on the history. This tickler system helps Dr. Brown remember all the steps he wishes to take for this particular patient. As he conducts his examination of Mr. Jones, he has his nurse check the other box that confirms he actually performed these examinations steps. He discusses the results of his examination with Mr. Jones and suggests a preliminary treatment plan. He explains to Mr. Jones that a copy of his final plan will be sent by e-mail to the patient at the same time it is sent to the primary care physician, and any further tests or follow-up visits will be scheduled at that time. Upon completing the examination and consultation, he reviews the automatically generated note, uses his stylus to indicate that he sees no need to dictate further information via the wireless voice-recognition system, and signs the note electronically. This signature automatically generates an e-prescription to Mr. Jones's pharmacy, codes the office visit, bills the insurance company, and sends a message to the front-desk worker of the amount to collect from Mr. Jones. In addition, a series of patient education handouts personalized for Mr. Jones are printed at the checkout desk and also sent as a PDF file to Mr. Jones's e-mail address. The system also self-generates an e-mail reminder to Mr. Jones to select a follow-up appointment time slot from the doctor's website. Mr. Jones says goodbye to Dr. Brown and his entire staff of two and heads to work [26].

Summary

Medical records management is essential to the delivery of high-quality health care. The amount of time and money invested in the current process, however, far exceeds the usefulness that it provides to busy specialists. To remain professionally successful and financially viable in the twenty-first century, urologists have to use every means at their disposal to improve the efficiency of record keeping and to speed up access to this information. Government and societal forces are pushing urologists inexorably toward EHR but certain major barriers must be overcome to increase the

momentum. For most urologists, the software selected will contribute less to successful implementation than will the physicians' willingness to adapt to a new process. Ultimately, the shift to interoperable EHR will result in significant overhead reductions, despite the near-term capital costs. Living in the information age means that affordable quality health care in the future will be a team effort between patients, their families, and all the providers and caregivers who are involved. Every member of the new expanded health care team requires immediate and often simultaneous access to patient information to contribute to solutions for health problems. All urologists should be developing a strategic plan to bring their practice into the age of electronic information quickly and economically.

References

[1] Edelstein L. Translation from the Greek, the Hippocratic oath: text, translation, and interpretation. Baltimore: Johns Hopkins Press; 1943.

[2] U.S. Department of Labor, Bureau of Labor Statistics. Occupational outlook handbook, 2004–2005 edition. (0*NET 29–2071.00). Available at: http://www.bls.gov/oco/ocos103.htm. Accessed April 30, 2005.

[3] Terry K. Exclusive survey—doctors and EHRs. Med Econ 2005;82:73.

[4] The business of urology survey of practice managers 2002. Baltimore (MD): American Urological Association; p. 7 [table 1.1].

[5] 2004 Health Policy Survey. Santa Ana (CA): Western Section AUA. 2004. p. 11.

[6] Babbitt N. Advancing initiatives for group practices. Medical Group Management Association Audio Conference; January 24, 2005. Englewood, CO.

[7] Survey of electronic health record trends and usage for 2004. Medical Records Institute; 2004 [table 5]. Available at: http://www.medrecinst.com/uploadedFiles/resources/EHR%20SURVEY%20RESULTS-2004-Web.pdf. Accessed April 30, 2005.

[8] The President's health information technology plan. Available at: www.whitehouse.gov/infocus/technology/economic_policy200404/chap3html. Accessed March 15, 2005.

[9] Brailer D. Advancing initiatives for group practices. Medical Group Management Association Audio Conference; January 24, 2005. Englewood, CO.

[10] Fraizer C. E-prescribing in clinical practice. J Med Practice Management 2004;20:148.

[11] Doyon C. Best practices in record completion. J Med Practice Management 2004;20:18.

[12] Robeznieks A. Adding performance data to EMR shows payoff. AMNews. December 27, 2004.

[13] U.S. healthcare provider I.T. spending. Health-Leaders Magazine. January 13, 2005.

[14] Chin T. Small practices fuel sales of EMR systems. AMNews. February 9, 2004.

[15] American College of Rheumatology. Electronic medical records for the physician's office. Available at: www.rheumatology.org. p. 31. Accessed February 28, 2005.

[16] Survey of electronic health record trends and usage for 2004. Medical Records Institute; 2004 [table 11]. Available at: http://www.medrecinst.com/uploadedFiles/resources/EHR%20SURVEY%20RESULTS-2004-Web.pdf. Accessed April 30, 2005.

[17] Pope C. Group practices identify, overcome EHR barriers. Connexion 2005;55(1):32.

[18] KLAS Enterprises. Top 20: 2004 best in KLAS. Available at: www.healthcomputing.com. KLAS Confidential Information. Accessed March 15, 2005.

[19] Miller S. Advancing initiatives for group practices. Medical Group Management Association Audio Conference; January 24, 2005. Englewood, CO.

[20] Cost. Survey for urology practices 2004 report based on 2003 data. Medical Group Management Association Audio Conference; January 24, 2004. Englewood, CO.

[21] Security rule manual HIPAA. A how-to implementation guide. Baltimore (MD): Gates, Moore & Company; 2003. p. 1.

[22] Quinn J. Lessons from the UK EMR: not exactly apples to apples. Healthleaders News. November 19, 2004.

[23] Tennant R. Advancing initiatives for group practices. Medical Group Management Association Audio Conference; January 24, 2005. Englewood, CO.

[24] HHS's health information technology efforts, GAO-04–991R. Washington (DC): Government Accounting Office. August 2004.

[25] Find a urologist. Available at: http://www.UrologyHealth.org/. Accessed April 30, 2005.

[26] Cap, Gemini, Ernst & Young. Evolving to a Connected Health Marketplace, Technology-Enabled Change in the US Health System. Available at: www.medrecinst.com. Accessed July 1, 2004.

ELSEVIER SAUNDERS

Urol Clin N Am 32 (2005) 285–290

UROLOGIC CLINICS of North America

Coding and Reimbursement: The Lifeline of the Urologist's Office

Stephanie N. Stinchcomb, CPC, CCS-P

*Practice Management Department, American Urological Association, 1000 Corporate Boulevard,
Linthicum, MD 21090, USA*

Coding rules and regulations change constantly, and this volume of *Urologic Clinics of North America* is not intended to be a coding and reimbursement course. Hopefully, all readers of this issue periodically send their staff (physicians and coders) to courses to learn the latest wrinkles in coding. Accurate coding depends on the information sources that the coding staff has available. A valuable and comprehensive compilation of many information resources is included at the end of this article.

According to the jointly sponsored *2003 Medical Group Management Association—American Urological Association Cost Survey for Urology Practices*, the mean cost of running urology offices, including medical liability insurance, employees' salaries, rent, utilities, supplies, and benefits, composes an average of 50.07% of office revenue (actual reimbursement of services, not gross charges) [1]. The only way to lower this number, the overhead, is to increase the efficiency and accuracy of billing operations.

M. Ray Painter, MD, president of Physician Reimbursement Systems, who consults for urology practices throughout the country, has stated that by learning and improving the coding and billing process, he has seen many offices increase revenue 5% to 15% a year. One old rule still applies, however: "If you did it, document it; if you document it, charge for it; if you didn't document it, you can't charge for it." With good documentation, proper coding and appropriate reimbursement follow.

Coding must be done correctly and ethically. According to the *Code of Ethics*, from the American Academy of Professional Coders (AAPC), "Members shall use only legal and ethical means in all professional dealings, and shall refuse to cooperate with or condone by silence, the actions of those who engage in fraudulent, deceptive or illegal acts" [2]. Coding and billing staff must have the reassurance that when a problem or error is discovered, the situation will be corrected, errors will be eliminated, and no one will be punished.

All offices must have policies that include

- An office compliance plan
- How to handle billing errors and how to correct them
- How to handle inquiries by patients

The urologists ultimately are responsible for any billing infractions. The name at the bottom of the Centers for Medicare and Medicaid Services (CMS) 1500 form belongs to the physician: physicians are responsible for what is on the bills they send, either solo practitioners, members of a large group, or those academic university practices. In an audit, it does not make any difference if someone claims to not know coding was being done in a particular way. The Office of the Inspector General does not allow ignorance as a defense. That is why urologists must be involved in the oversight of coding staff. Their names at the bottom of the form mean that they are the ones the agents from the Office of the Inspector General visit if there is a problem. If urologists and their practices follow the rules, they have nothing to fear.

E-mail address: w.f.gee@att.net

0094-0143/05/$ - see front matter © 2005 Elsevier Inc. All rights reserved.
doi:10.1016/j.ucl.2005.04.006

It is, therefore, imperative for offices to keep current on

- New coding directives
- New guidelines
- Medicare bundling edits (*National Correct Coding Initiative* [*NCCI*])
- New carrier coverage determinations
- Quarterly drug payment updates
- Yearly changes to *Current Procedural Terminology* (*CPT*)
- Twice yearly changes to *International Classification of Diseases, Ninth Revision* (*ICD-9*) diagnosis terminology

History of *Current Procedural Terminology*: the language of coding

Medical coding is a language. Billing is built on trust: a *CPT* procedure code coupled with an *ICD-9* diagnosis code is sent in and money is sent back [3,4]. *CPT* translates the service provided to the patient into dollars, and the reason for the medical service into a language that insurance carriers can understand. The development of medical coding began in 1966 with publication of the first American Medical Association (AMA) *CPT* nomenclature book. The first edition of the *CPT* contained surgical procedures with limited sections on medicine, radiology, and laboratory services. In 1983, the CMS (formerly Health Care Financing Administration) adopted *CPT* nomenclature as part of the *Healthcare Common Procedure Coding System* (*HCPCS*), known as hick-picks [5]. *CPT* codes were required to report services for Part B of the Medicare program. In October 1986, CMS mandated that state Medicaid agencies use *HCPCS* codes. In July 1987, CMS required that *CPT* codes be used to report outpatient hospital procedures. Through the Health Insurance Portability and Accessibility Act of 1996 (HIPAA), *CPT* codes became the national standard for reporting services to insurance carriers in 2000.

Keeping up to date—resources

It is imperative that coding staff work with valid and timely coding tools. Just as surgeons cannot operate without the proper instruments, office billing staff cannot do their job without up-to-date resources. Manuals must be purchased every year to ensure appropriate coding of medical claims and eliminate the denials of inappropriately billed claims. The absolute minimum reference sources that must be purchased new every year include

- *CPT*
- *ICD-9, Clinical Modification* (*ICD-9-CM*)
- *HCPCS*, which lists national Medicare codes, to report medical services, supplies, drugs, and certain procedures not defined by *CPT*.
- *NCCI*, which is essential in billing claims for Medicare beneficiaries. *NCCI* is updated quarterly and includes edits established by AdminaStar Federal, the Medicare contractor for the edits. These edits tell which *CPT* codes can be billed together, which are reimbursed separately, and which cannot be billed together [6].

Grace period eliminated

In 2005, CMS eliminated the grace period for Medicare claims. In the past, physicians' offices and carriers had 90 days to implement new codes or eliminate deleted codes before claims would face denial. With the elimination of the grace period, when a code is effective, it must be implemented in the coding vocabulary. *CPT* codes are updated every January 1; *ICD-9-CM* diagnosis codes are updated April 1 and October 1; and *HCPCS* codes are updated either January 1 or July 1. Medicare reimbursement in the form of relative values are updated each January.

Hiring essential staff

Once the resources are available, they are only as good as the people using them. Hiring staff that is knowledgeable of the coding rules and government regulations and who have a sense of the importance of ethical and accurate coding is vital. Understanding coding takes years of application, research, skill, and a basic drive to get the job done correctly. Ideal coders should understand how to use all the coding resources, be self-motivated, and be willing to investigate and research when the information provided does not sound right. When a claim is denied unjustly, staff must be diligent in pursuing the payment of the claim through appropriate appeal processes.

Certifications

There are two national organizations that certify individuals as professional coders:

- AAPC. This is the only organization devoted solely to the advancement of coding.

Individuals can become a member of the AAPC but do not have to become certified. The AAPC has a designation of certified professional coder (CPC). CPC is a coding certification for office-based coding. The dues are nominal and credentialing must be maintained yearly by attending conferences, meetings, and seminars to keep current on important coding issues.

- The American Health Information Management Association. This organization supports coding certification in the designation of certified coding specialist–physician based.

Self-policing—the internal audit process

Many offices find that an internal audit process helps in billing appropriate claims. A peer review audit helps physicians to self-police. These audits can be performed a twice a year to maintain adequate coding and documentation of evaluation and management services. Several charts from each physician are reviewed by colleagues to determine proper documentation and if the appropriate level of evaluation and management service was chosen and billed. This is an excellent educational opportunity to make sure all are kept on their toes and do not become complacent in the choice of appropriate level of evaluation and management service. Doing this in an informal group setting is most educational.

Basic coding resources for every urology practice

Coding and reimbursement is a complex and inexact science. Sometimes there is no right answer. Knowing all of the resources and where to look for the answers, however, ensures the best possible outcome.

American Urological Association services for coding and reimbursement

The AUA offers many services to assist physicians and their staff members to code claims to Medicare and other third-party insurance companies accurately and efficiently.

Coding tips for urologist offices

Each year the AUA provides *Coding Tips* on line as a free service. This informative guide offers education on new *CPT*, *ICD-9*, and *HCPCS* codes. It is an important resource for physicians and billing and coding staff. The chart of most frequently billed urology *CPT* codes has been improved with conversion to an electronic Medicare fee calculator based on Medicare region. When accessing this chart, select only the Medicare region or state to automatically generate a list of the 100 most frequently billed Medicare allowables for a practice. This is a helpful tool to assure proper payment from Medicare carriers.

Coding hotline

The AUA has CPCs on staff to assist with difficult coding problems and coverage issues. Subscribers to the Practice Managers' Network have unlimited free access to this service. Questions from nonsubscribers are answered for a nominal charge. There are several ways to submit specific coding questions: by telephone (866-746-4282), fax (410-689-3907), or e-mail (codinghotline@auanet.org). Operative reports, explanation of benefits, and other documentation and correspondence should accompany coding inquiries between practices and payers. Make sure all patient information has been deleted to comply with HIPAA regulations. To subscribe to the Practice Managers' Network, call 866-742-4282 for an application.

AUA Coding Today

This is a valuable on-line resource to assist in finding appropriate *CPT/ICD-9-CM/HCPCS*, state-specific Medicare payment information, global periods, and bundling edits. The AUA, in conjunction with Physicians Reimbursement Systems, has developed this useful tool. To sign up, go to www.auacodingtoday.com.

Coding education

Because coding rules are changing continually, even the best coders must strive to stay on top of all the new coding and payment rules affecting practices. By investing in their continuing education each year, practices will see a difference in accuracy and in reimbursements. The AUA offers comprehensive sessions on coding for evaluation and management services and urology procedural services held at regional seminars around the country.

New Current Procedural Terminology codes

Recommendations for new urologic *CPT* codes should be submitted by mail to Chairman, Coding and Reimbursement Committee, AUA, Reimbursement Systems Manager, American Urological Association, 1000 Corporate Boulevard, Linthicum, Maryland 21090, or by fax to 410-689-3907.

The AUA Government Affairs Department presents recommendations for new *CPT* codes to the AUA coding and reimbursement committee at their semiannual meeting to determine if the recommendation meets the following criteria for a new *CPT* code:

- Its technology is FDA approved.
- It is proved efficacious in peer-reviewed literature.
- It is an accepted or recognized procedure anticipated to become a standard service/practice.

Coding essentials—updated every year!

Whether or not urology practices consist of one physician or are a multispecialty group, urologists and the billing staff need specific resources for everyday use. Practices should renew these four coding books every year:

- *CPT*—this reference guide is an essential tool for urology practices and lists all of the current physician procedural and evaluation and management codes necessary for correct coding.
- *ICD-9-CM*—*Diseases Tabular List (Volume 1)* and *Diseases Alphabetical Index (Volume 2)*, which list all the diagnosis codes used by physicians. If practices do hospital billing, they also need the *ICD-9 Procedural Code*, which lists all *ICD-9-CM* hospital procedural codes.
- *HCPCS*
- *Medicare RBRVS: The Physician's Guide*, which is a guide to relative values for all *HCPCS* and *CPT* codes

Order these books from the AMA at 800-621-8335 or Ingenix at 877-464-3649.

These four publications are a small investment and provide invaluable information. Renewed annually, they save hours of miscoding, denied claims, and lost reimbursements. These books come in various formats: hardbound, softbound, computerized disk, and magnetic tape. It is important that tools fit the methods of billing; therefore, it may be cost effective to buy a computerized version.

National Correct Coding Initiative *coding edits*

This is an essential tool for urology offices that bill services for the Medicare population. The *NCCI* edits are maintained through CMS's contractor, AdminaStar Federal. The *NCCI* edits outline comprehensive and component code pairs for billing Medicare claims. The AUA offers a *NCCI* supplement in the January, April, July, and October issues of the AUA's *Health Policy Brief,* which lists code bundling edits specifically for urology. The federal government's National Technical Information Service offers the complete *National Correct Coding Policy Manual in Comprehensive Code Sequence for Part B Medicare Carriers* for all edits for a nominal fee. Order this publication by calling 800-363-2068 or visiting www.ntis.gov/product/correct-coding.htm. *NCCI* edits also are available free of charge by accessing the CMS Web site, www.cms.hhs.gov/physicians/cciedits. AUACodingToday.com also lists all NCCI edits.

If edits are found that are inappropriate, contact the AUA Government Affairs Department at 410-689-3780. The edits will be presented to CMS and AdminaStar for reconsideration.

Coding books, newsletters, and software

The following resources assist offices in understanding *CPT* coding, Medicare payment policy, and the national Medicare Fee Schedule for all procedures. This list is for informational purposes only and does not carry AUA endorsement.

- *Coding Companion for Urology–Nephrology* (formerly *Coding Illustrated, Genitourinary System*), a book developed by Ingenix, which provides an illustrative and layman's explanation of all the genitourinary *CPT* codes. Also listed with each code are the most commonly associated *ICD-9* codes and billable *HCPCS* level II codes for outpatient services. To order, call 877-464-3649.
- *Coding News*, a newsletter devoted to *ICD-9* coding issues. To order, call 800-825-7421.
- *Part B News*, a newsletter dedicated to Medicare policy and reimbursement news. To order, call 877-602-3835. (Note: AUA members receive a discount when subscribing to this publication.)
- *Urology Coder's Pink Sheets*, a newsletter specifically dealing with urology coding issues. To order, call 877-602-3835. (Note: AUA members receive a discount when subscribing to this publication.)
- *CPT Assistant*, an AMA newsletter that provides articles on coding and answers to common coding questions. To order, call 800-621-8335.

- Electronic billing resources can help if practices submit claims electronically. Medicare carriers offer a software package at cost that allows printing and viewing claims in a Medicare standard format. For more information, contact the carrier and ask about the *American National Standards Institute ASCX12835 Electronic Claims Remittance Form* (PC-Print-V). (Visit cms.hhs.gov/contacts/incardir.asp for a telephone and Web site listing of Medicare carriers' medical directors.)

American Academy of Professional Coders

The AAPC is one of the nation's largest medical coding organizations. For membership or certification information, call 800-626-2633 or visit www.aapc.com.

American Health Information Management Association

The American Health Information Management Association is another organization promoting coding through certification and membership. For more information, call 312-233-1100 or visit www.ahima.org.

Medicare informational resources

Medicare—Centers for Medicare and Medicaid Services

There is a Web site provided through CMS for physicians at www.cms.hhs.gov/physicians. This is a physician resource page that includes all necessary information, including *NCCI*, fee schedule information, drug payments, and so forth.

Medicare carrier advisory committees

The CMS mandates that all carriers maintain an advisory committee made up of physicians from every specialty to allow open communications among providers and payers. This effort has been successful in many states in clarifying local coding and reimbursement issues. Carriers do not employ these practicing urologists and other physicians; rather, carrier advisory committees (CACs) serve as contact points to voice urologic concerns brought forward from providers and payers.

Urologist representatives on each state CAC and the Medicare medical directors are listed at www.auanet.org/coding/codingtips/caclist.cfm. The AUA includes these urology CAC members on a committee that meets at the AUA annual meeting. These urologists are nominated by state medical or urologic societies and appointed to serve on the Medicare CAC.

Centers for Medicare and Medicaid Services training courses

CMS, which is responsible for the Medicare program, now offers several on-line Medicare training courses. CMS also offers other training courses for physician staff at remote locations. For details about these courses and how to access them, visit cms.hhs.gov/medlearn/.

Centers for Medicare and Medicaid Services regional offices

The United States is divided into 10 CMS regions. Medicare carriers (for physician and hospital services) are insurance companies that bid and are awarded government contracts by CMS to provide claims processing to Medicare beneficiaries within a specified area. These contractors report to the CMS regional offices and to the national CMS office in Baltimore. The regional offices also award durable medical equipment numbers. For reference, the addresses of the 10 CMS regional offices are listed at this Web site: cms.hhs.gov/about/regions/professionals.asp.

Medicare Part B carriers

Each Medicare carrier has it own Web site to update providers of new local coverage determinations or any new updated Medicare information. Go to www.cms.hhs.gov/contacts/incardir.asp for a list of Medicare Part B carriers.

References

[1] 2003 Medical Group Management Association—American Urological Association cost survey for urology practices.
[2] American Academy of Professional Coders. Code of ethics.
[3] Current procedural terminology (CPT). American Medical Association; 2004.
[4] International classification of diseases, ninth revision (ICD-9).
[5] Healthcare common procedure coding system.
[6] National correct coding initiatives.

Informational Web sites

Centers for Medicare & Medicaid Services. cms.hhs.gov.
Ambulatory Surgical Center Information. www.cms.hhs.gov/suppliers/asc/.

Advanced Beneficiary Notice. cms.hhs.gov/medlearn/ refguide.asp.

Clinical laboratory information. www.cms.hhs.gov/ suppliers/clinlab/default.asp (laboratory testing).

Coverage determinations—local and national. www. cms.hhs.gov/coverage/.

CPT utilization statistical files. cms.hhs.gov/statistics/ feeforservice/default.asp.

Drug payments—quarterly update. www.cms.hhs.gov/ providers/drugs/.

Durable medical equipment information. www.cms. hhs.gov/suppliers/dmepos.

Evaluation and management documentation guidelines. cms.hhs.gov/medlearn/emdoc.asp.

Fee schedule look up. www.cms.hhs.gov/physicians/ mpfsapp/step0.asp.

Healthcare common procedural coding. www.cms.hhs. gov/medicare/hcpcs/.

ICD-9-CM diagnosis coding. www.cms.hhs.gov/ paymentsystems/icd9/default.asp.

ICD-9-CM official guidelines for *ICD-9-CM* coding. www.cdc.gov/nchs/data/icd9/icdguide.pdf.

ICD-10 proposed system. www.cms.hhs.gov/ paymentsystems/icd9/icd10.asp.

Physicians' Regulatory Issues Team. cms.hhs.gov/ physicians/prit/.

HCPCS coding. cms.hhs.gov/medicare/hcpcs.

Medicare carriers. cms.hhs.gov/contacts/incardir.asp.

Medicare carrier manual. cms.hhs.gov/manuals/14_car/ 3btoc.asp Part III (Physician Billing) Coding Guidelines Chapter 15.——

Medicare regional offices—durable. cms.hhs.gov/contacts/ incardir.asp Medical Equipment.

Medicare regional offices. www.cms.hhs.gov/about/ regions/professionals.asp.

Medicare learning network—interactive medicare coding and billing training for staff www.cms.hhs.gov/ medlearn/.

MEDLEARN matters—articles on new Medicare issues. /www.cms.hhs.gov/medlearn/matters/.

Medicare participating physician directory. www1. medicare.gov/Physician/Search/PhysicianSearch.asp.

National correct coding initiative. www.cms.hhs.gov/ physicians/cciedits.

Program manuals, transmittals and memos. cms.hhs.gov/ manuals/default.asp.

Quarterly provider updates. www.cms.hhs.gov/ providerupdate/.

RVUs. cms.hhs.gov/physicians/pfs/.

Skilled nursing facility information. www.cms.hhs.gov/ providers/snfpps/.

UPIN numbers for referring physicians. /upin.ecare. com or cms.hhs.gov/providers/enrollment/upin/ Upinsrc.asp#P0_0.

Searchable *ICD-9-CM* database. www.eicd.com/EICDMain. htm or www.icd9coding1.com/flashcode/home.jsp.

American Medical Association. www.ama-assn.org.

CPT information and education. www.ama-assn.org/ ama/pub/category/3884.html.

FDA. www.fda.gov.

List of drugs and corresponding national drug codes. www.fda.gov/cder/ndc/.

Office of Inspector General—compliance guidelines, provider exclusion lists. oig.hhs.gov.

Database of drugs, uses, generic/brand names. my. webmd.com/medical_information/drug_and_herb/ default.htm.

On-line medical dictionary. medical-dictionary.com/.

Information on surgeries/medical terminology. www. google.com/.

Medical articles. www.nlm.nih.gov/medlineplus/.

ELSEVIER
SAUNDERS

Urol Clin N Am 32 (2005) 291–297

**UROLOGIC
CLINICS**
of North America

Strategic Planning and Budgeting

Nick A. Fabrizio, PhD[a,b,*], Kenneth T. Hertz[b]

[a]Department of Family Medicine, Upstate Medical University, SUNY at Syracuse, Syracuse, NY, USA
[b]Medical Group Management Association, Health Care Consulting Group, Alexandria, LA, USA

Medical groups must take the time to inventory their current short-term strategies, measure their success, and make course corrections in a proactive methodologic process. At the same time, it is important to develop a long-term strategy for market share and profitability. The strategic planning process is a way for groups to satisfy current and future needs while solidifying the group's mission, vision, and harmony.

Budgeting is an integral part of a medical practice's long- and short-term planning processes. Budget development requires a deep and thorough understanding of a practice's infrastructure, operations, and processes. In addition to the creation of financial goals, the budget process ensures that the management team and physician leadership continue to be well informed regarding a practice's health.

Strategic planning

To succeed, groups must have an effective strategic planning process in place. Prioritizing and framing a strategic planning initiative usually fall under the responsibility of an administrator and a group's leadership. The need for planning may come about through changes in the external environment, including regulatory requirements, or through an internal process initiated by physicians, staff, or management.

An administrator's overall role in strategic planning is that of coordination, initiation, and implementation [1]. Some believe that although the strategic planning process must be initiated, coordinated, and implemented, the real value and benefit of the process is the facilitation by a qualified professional who has a background in data gathering and analysis, pattern matching, and organizational and group development. Facilitators must be objective in their assessment of the issues and skillful in developing relationships with key personnel to obtain accurate and complete information. They then need to frame the issues, develop themes, and help the group facilitate the process of moving the organization to decision making. Often, leaders or administrators of a group are too close to the organizations to be able to develop independent judgments about the issues. They also may lack objectivity that leads others to feel comfortable sharing their true feelings about the current state of affairs or future needs. Outside or independent facilitators often are seen as persons that others can confide in with the goal of sharing confidential information for process improvements.

The importance of strategic planning

The majority of decisions in operating today's medical groups falls under the philosophies of "If it ain't broke—don't fix it"; management by crisis; or fighting today's fire. Groups rarely spend time thinking about strategy defined as their role in the community; role in the department; staffing and physician needs, including recruitment; or acquisition and divestiture strategies. Medical groups must take the time to inventory their current short-term strategies, measure their success, and make course corrections in a proactive methodologic process.

It also is important to distinguish between strategic plans, which are long-term in nature,

---

* Corresponding author. Department of Family Medicine, Upstate Medical University, 475 Irving Avenue, Suite 200, Syracuse, NY 13210.
 E-mail address: fabrizin@upstate.edu (N.A. Fabrizio).

0094-0143/05/$ - see front matter © 2005 Elsevier Inc. All rights reserved.
doi:10.1016/j.ucl.2005.03.010

from short-term action plans that are designed to implement the strategies [2]. Administrators must keep track of long-term plans and the action plans that are needed to accomplish those objectives. In the strategic planning process, the group often can determine the long-term objectives and brainstorm ideas and strategies needed to accomplish those objectives; however, it is critical that the leadership take the selected long-term action plans back to the middle managers and staff to determine how realistic some of the group's current capabilities are and to identify areas of weakness for external support. For instance, if a group determines the need to implement an electronic medical record (EMR), the strategic planning process may have identified the need, outlined the process from the request for proposal to vendor selection to implementation, and assigned a leader to the project. When this plan is brought back to the end users and middle managers, however, the group may uncover additional information vital to developing the long-term plan, such as how many users can be on the system at any given time, the need to upgrade any of the current computers, the need for some of the staff, who are and computer savvy, to have additional training, and so forth. These all are factors that determine effective implementation.

Determining a group's readiness

How can a group know if it is ready for a strategic planning process? There are several strategic questions to consider:

- Is there a high staff or physician turnover ratio?
- What kinds of services should the group provide?
- Is the practice losing market share to competitors?
- Is the practice having a difficult time retaining good administrators or managers?
- Is there a group culture that is difficult to define?
- Is the decision-making process led by strong governance, or are decisions made based on who complains the loudest or most frequently?
- Do people in the organization know and understand the mission, vision, and values?
- Can members of the group define the top two business or strategic initiatives?
- What resources will be required in the future and where will they come from?

When a group commits to the strategic planning process, it is helpful to have preretreat meetings with all of the staff, physicians, and leaders separately and then jointly to discuss what they believe their current mission, vision, and values are. This may take a series of meetings, but these meetings should focus on refining the current mission, vision, and values, because this is going to be the foundation of the strategic planning process. Once the planning process is begun, the group's current and future goals are compared with the group's agreed-upon mission, vision, and values. This aids in promoting group buy-in and commitment.

Identify major issues threatening the group

Part of the planning process involves determining if there are any major factors threatening the group. Some of these questions include:

- Are any physicians planning on retiring in the next 12 months?
- When are physicians planning on retiring or leaving the group?
- Are the staff or physicians unhappy about their compensation system?
- Is the current rent or lease arrangement about to expire or are is there new property management?
- Is there a major piece of medical equipment that needs to be replaced?
- Is the practice implementing an EMR?
- Is the practice recruiting new physicians?

These factors should be discussed and framed during the strategic planning process to develop a project timeline to navigate through these issues. Again, the success of this step is achieved through a careful preplanning process in which the facilitator and administrator can begin to gather data from individual and group meetings.

Having the right people present and participating

A key to success is having the appropriate people present and participating in the strategic planning process. There must be enough time allocated in the leaders' schedules to make the process a high enough priority to get people's attention. Ascertain if there are the right people in the organization ready to move forward rather than relish on past successes or the way things were. Once it is determined that the right people are in the organization, create an environment of action, risk taking, and tolerance. Employees must be energized by the mission, vision, and short- and long-term goals and must be active participants in moving the organization forward.

Strengths, weaknesses, opportunities, and threats assessment

As part of the preretreat process, many facilitators ask participants individually to list strengths, weaknesses, opportunities, and threats. This information can be tabulated and organized by theme and brought to the retreat process for group discussion. By doing this, the organization can get a more comprehensive idea of how individuals rate the group on these items. Skillful facilitators then can get a group to buy in to developing some themes and begin a process to identify and prioritize the issues.

The major steps of the planning process can be summarized by finding answers to the following questions:

1. Where is the practice now and where does it want to be in the future?
2. What is happening in the external and internal environments that is preventing achievement of the objectives?
3. What do the members of the group and employees think will help the practice succeed?
4. How does the practice get to where it wants to go?
5. Does your plan have clear timelines and delineated responsibilities?

The first step is to review the current status of the organization and identify the mission, vision, values, and current beliefs. The group also must identify the current problems of the organization and define where it wants to be positioned in the future.

The second step is to gather data on where the group is in the market and what the external environment looks like. Issues related to this phase include regulatory requirements; insurance changes; the competitive landscape; relationships with other specialists, primary care physicians, and hospitals; and so forth. The internal environment also must be addressed by looking at the skills and competencies of the physicians, administrators, managers, and employees. The group's culture and decision-making process also must be addressed to better determine the ability to

respond to the next steps in the plan, including major issues related to redirecting the group's business plan.

The third step is to ask employees, physicians, and patients their opinions of where the group is now and to identify services they would like to have. The goal of this step is to hear from constituents and have a process that respects, appreciates, and documents their views and opinions. This step also validates the importance of everyone's role in the process, which serves as a catalyst for change.

The fourth step is deciding where to go and how to get there. This is where to begin developing a plan that is related to step five, which is active action planning. In this step, gather data and list clear and specific action plans that detail what the group wants to do, how it is going to do it, and by when; assign a person to each action plan. These plans are shared with employees and group members so they can see where their opinions relate to the plans (part of group buy-in) and help refine the plans and make course corrections. This helps ensure short-term and long-term success.

Example of a strategic decision: hiring another physician to join a group

The group is unanimous in this decision, although they are cautious in moving forward because of what happened with the previous two physicians recruited into the group. One of these physicians separated from the group because of quality concerns and the other left within 10 months because of unhappiness with his quality of life outside of the office. The group discussed the importance in hiring for fit and making sure the candidates are exposed to community offerings.

Action steps
Define expectations and recruitment strategy. The position is defined better to match candidate to current and future strategic plans. The goals of this recruitment effort led to the following action plan:

- Recruiting a female physician 40 years of age or younger—female preferred if hired within the next 2 years
- Permitting a full-time or part-time position
- Recruiting someone willing to accept partnership track responsibilities
- Recruiting someone who is hard working for inpatient, outpatient, nursing home, and house calls; need to develop a job description

- Starting advertising in next 6 months
- Recruitment beginning after advertising by month 8
- Advertising in hospitals, journals, local newspapers, select city newspapers, and state medical societies
- Awareness of and actively managing transition issues; if a practice hires a female physician, an immediate decision needs to be made regarding current nurse practitioner

A compensation package needs to be determined. The current financial position of the practice and cash flow are factors that need further attention. Various issues need to be explored, such as

- Offering a small ($90,000) base salary guarantee with productivity incentives built in
- Offering a medium to small base salary, which is reduced yearly with productivity incentives
- Offering productivity-based compensation; this option, however, will produce only a few interested applicants, unless they already are within the community or join from another group in the current catchment areas
- Asking if the hospital can subsidize or employ the physician

Responsibility

The administrator explores these options, documents progress on each, develops a timeline for each responsibility, and shares updates with the group at monthly practice meetings.

Time frame

This task will be completed between October 2004 to December 2004.

Conclusion: communicate the plan

Once a plan is documented and revised with clear action plans, timelines, and responsible individuals listed for those plans, the action plans should be shared with the group and employees. The strategic plans should be updated monthly and posted in a place, such as the break room or lunchroom, so that the employees and physicians can track the plans, timelines, and progress. These displays also are referred to as mapping or storyboards and are common in industries outside of health care. The goal of the strategic planning process is to develop realistic plans that have been reviewed actively by all staff and agreed to by the

group's leadership. These plans also should be discussed at staff meetings and physician meetings routinely to keep members informed while soliciting comments on these plans and future plans. Soliciting feedback and actively engaging all members of the group help them feel connected while serving as the basis for future strategic plans.

Budgeting

One of the major components of an organization's planning efforts is the process of budgeting. Although there is discussion in the field concerning the overall value of budgeting to a medical group, the literature abounds with anecdotal information regarding best practices of successful groups and their intensity and focus on the budgeting process. For a group to be successful, it must have access to information to assist in decision making, organizational control, providing data for monitoring and negotiating managed care contracts, and assisting management and physician leadership in overall financial planning. Budgeting can provide this assistance.

Why budget?

The process of budgeting in a medical organization follows closely that of strategic and operational planning. Once the details of future operations are articulated, the group needs to determine the requirements and availability of resources to reach the stated goals. The budgeting discipline requires a clear understanding of the goals to be achieved, the strategies and tactics to be employed, and the external environment that serves as a backdrop for the plan.

Various organizational components are required to attain a high level of communication and cooperation to create organizational financial goals and objectives. The process provides the opportunity for all levels of an organization to participate, come together, and arrive at the final budget. A properly constructed budget, one built from the bottom up, engenders buy-in at all organizational levels and helps ensure a sense of personal responsibility for achieving the goals.

Operationally, once the budget is created, reviewed, and approved, it provides a benchmark for an organization to compare financial results on a periodic basis throughout the year, to evaluate the cause of variances from the benchmark, and to make timely operational revisions as necessary. Further, under the proper guidance of an administrator, the budget serves as a motivator for staff to strive for agreed-on financial goals and as a guide for budgeted expenditures. The absence of a budget creates a situation suggested in the admonition, "If you don't know where you are going, there is a good chance you won't get there!"

What are the components of a budget?

This article focuses on what often is called a comprehensive or master budget. There are simpler approaches that are less inclusive but operationally not as helpful. A comprehensive budget generally consists of revenue and expense, cash flow, acquisition or sale of assets, and detailed discussions and projections regarding these areas.

Revenue budget

A revenue budget is developed using external and internal data sets. Practices review external environmental issues, including the local market, changing demographics, the local economy, and the reimbursement environment correlating to the specific specialty.

Internal data review includes historical payer mix, analysis of patients by age and sex, current procedural terminology procedural volume analysis, and pertinent trending. In addition, decisions about changes in provider practice patterns, clinic capacity, the addition or deletion (through retirement, resignation, termination, or slowdown) of providers and midlevel providers, and new or deleted product lines all must be considered in developing a revenue budget.

In most cases, a budget is developed on a cash basis (discussed later in this article); therefore, monthly revenue budget figures are actual revenue anticipated that month rather than gross charge figures (Alternatively, there are practices, more financially mature, that are preferable for providing monthly gross revenue figures with adjustments calculated based on historical information and projected payer mix. Both alternatives are acceptable).

Although the simple approach to developing the revenue (or expense) budget may be to take the previous year's figures and increase it by a percentage based on certain expectations of growth (incremental increases), best practices supports a zero-based approach that provides realistic and defensible budget forecasting, or a newer approach, activity-based costing. (Zero-based budgeting uses historical data as a reference point but develops future projections from scratch using multiple data sets and informational resources. The zero-based budgeting approach is more comprehensive and time-consuming than the incremental approach. Activity cost-based budgets focus on a per-service cost and tie revenue and expense directly to projected levels of activity within a practice.)

Expense budget

The development of the expense budget is based on the behavior of costs in various patterns. This article focuses on fixed and variable costs.

Fixed costs may be understood as those costs that do not vary with patient volume. In other words, costs that continue day in and day out: rent, utilities, most personnel, malpractice insurance, and so forth. These costs are affected not by the number of patients but by contracts or leadership decisions in the planning process.

Variable costs are activity based and reflective of patient volume and production levels. These costs include medical supplies, disposables, laboratory testing costs, and so forth.

In order that a viable and realistic expense budget is developed, practices must review and understand the behavior of each cost (expense) category. The questions must be asked, "Is this cost fixed or variable?" and "How will it behave?" Once answered, expense budget projections may be developed based on a combination of historical information, productivity and activity projections, and an understanding of pertinent contractual obligations.

Although the handling of physician compensation varies significantly from practice to practice and often depends on the corporate structure and tax basis, it is critical that an expense budget is developed with timely and adequate input from the physicians. This step ties directly to the development of the revenue budget. Physicians must understand the correlation between revenue generation and compensation. An expense budget must reflect the compensation expectations of the physicians within the resources available from their production.

Practices will find it useful to secure input, particularly in the development of the expense budget, as they assist in the financial control process through organizational buy-in.

Operating budget

An operating budget combines revenue and expense budgets for an overall picture of a practice's financial operating goals. It is this budget that is used as a management tool to ensure focus and adherence to the predetermined plan, to provide a basis for measurement of variances from the plan, and to serve as a foundation for the development of alternative and course correction plans.

The operating budget includes cash and non-cash items; for the purpose of budgeting cash flow, the noncash items must be removed from the budget. This function generally falls to a practice accountant or a practice's manager.

Capital budget

As part of the strategic planning process, practices develop long- and short-term projections of capital expenditures. These may include office modifications or construction or equipment pur-chase, either new or upgrades. Often neglected in practices' planning is the programmed updating of computer network equipment. Failure to ade-quately plan for this may result in emergent needs for borrowing capital and a sudden increase in cash outflow. Thoughtful, thorough budgeting prepares practices financially for such occurrences and provides contingency plans for unforeseen situations.

Cash versus accrual basis accounting

The difference between cash and accrual basis of accounting must be understood for the de-velopment of useful financial and management reports and tools. Simply put, the cash basis records income when cash is received and records expenses when cash is spent, whereas the accrual basis of accounting records revenue when it is earned and records expenses when they are in-curred. It is this second method that falls within the guidelines prescribed by generally accepted accounting principles [3].

A better picture of actual operating results is provided by the accrual method, but it does not necessarily provide the needed detail in operating cash flow. If a budget is prepared on a complete accrual basis and practices maintain their books on a cash basis, the actual monthly results vary significantly from the budget. It is for this reason that many practices monitor results on a quarterly basis to balance the distortion that may occur between the cash basis results and the usefulness of the data.

How to use the budget and related financial statements

As discussed previously, a budget serves as an internal benchmark to measure progress toward stated financial goals. Formatting of financial statements, for example an income statement with detailed budgets, is done on a monthly or quarterly basis and includes actual results for the time period, the budgeted amount for the same time period on an account-by-account basis, and, in many cases, a comparison to the same period in the previous year. Management is asked to prepare a variance report and to address discrepancies between actual performance and the budget and previous year. Too often, practices do not conduct this thorough variance analysis, and problems remain unidentified in the early and repairable stages, instead transforming into a crisis.

The balance sheet is another financial state-ment, a favorite of accountants, but, in most cases, not reviewed heavily in a medical practice. As a function of budgeting, the complete budget-ing process includes a look at a practice's balance sheet at the beginning of the year and a projection of the balance sheet at the end of the year based on cash flow, projections of the practice's resour-ces regarding payables, efficiency in receivables, abilities adequately projecting capital needs, and debt management.

As do other industries, medical practices rely heavily on cash flow for survival; as such, the cash flow statement is a critical document requiring review and analysis on a monthly basis. This statement often is called the source and use of funds statement. In this document, practices capture the cash inflow and outflow and provide projections to management as to whether or not there are sufficient financial resources for operat-ing and capital expenditures.

In effect, the budget and related financial statements become a critical component of a prac-tice's vital signs. A practice's accountant, man-agement team, and physician leadership should check them on a monthly basis. As discussed previously, variances must be reviewed and ana-lyzed with consideration given to those caused by accrual versus cash basis. Management's report should be written and presented to physician leadership before monthly meetings, and adequate time at the start of shareholder or board meetings should be provided for thorough review. The theory of no surprises must prevail. A practice's future depends on it.

Not only can a budget be used for financial review but, given its applicability to and correla-tion with practice operational statistics, the bud-get is a useful tool for measuring operational efficiencies and goal achievement.

The comparison of actual results to a thoughtfully prepared budget is an invaluable tool for management decision making. Financial and operational decisions can be set against a backdrop of hard data and performance results, rather than conjecture and hypothesis. When purchasing new equipment, adding a new staff member, or purchasing new supplies, the data available from actual to budget comparisons enable informed decision making and serve as a basis for financial control within the organization.

Summary

Budgeting is an integral part of a medical practice's long- and short-term planning processes. It provides a focus and a pricetag for an operational plan. The budgeting process promotes organizational teamwork and communication and assists in the development of well-articulated and time-sensitive goals. Budget development requires a deep and thorough understanding of a practice's infrastructure, operations, and processes. In addition to the creation of financial goals, the budget process ensures that the management team and physician leadership continue to be well informed regarding a practice's health.

References

[1] Bracker J. The historic development of the strategic management concept. Acad Manage Rev 1980;5: 219–24.
[2] Strombeck R. The strategic planning process: a guide for health care managers. Laguna Niguel (California): Healthcare Education Associates; 1992.
[3] Keagy B, Thomas M. Essentials of physician practice management. San Francisco: Jossey-Bass; 2004.

ELSEVIER SAUNDERS

Urol Clin N Am 32 (2005) 299–308

UROLOGIC CLINICS of North America

Marketing Your Urologic Practice—Ethically, Effectively, and Economically

Neil Baum, MD

Tulane University School of Medicine, 3525 Prytania, Suite 614, New Orleans, LA 70115, USA

If urologists find they are suffering from burnout and are not enjoying the practice of medicine as much as in the past; if they have a contracting population base; if they are receiving fewer referrals from colleagues than 2 years ago; if their practices have lost significant income with the new Medicare reimbursements for luteinizing hormone–releasing hormone agonists; or if managed care has moved existing patients to another health care provider, then this article is for them. It can help them create the kind of practice they want, target a desirable patient population, and get more of a handle on their business. All these goals can be attained by learning how to market a practice effectively, efficiently, and economically.

But some say they do not have the extra capital to invest in a marketing program. Effective marketing does not mean hiring a high-priced consultant and creating a five-color brochure with a snappy logo. Effective marketing means taking extraordinary care of existing patients, which can be done simply and economically.

The practice of urology has changed drastically and, like it or not, the importance of a marketing component to practices has become more important than ever before. It is important to have superb clinical skills and be able to implement the latest technology to treat urologic diseases. It also is important to learn how to market and promote practices ethically. Urologists who do not understand basic marketing principles as they relate to practice promotion are in danger of becoming ineffective healers. In contrast, those urologists who maintain a high level of clinical skill and marketing skills will find themselves equipped to practice medicine in an ever-changing environment.

The four pillars of marketing success

Successful urology practices have four components:

1. The patients who already are in the practice
2. The capacity to attract new patients
3. A motivated staff to take care of those patients
4. Excellent communication with referring physicians and other health care professionals

These four components are just like the poles supporting a tent: remove any one of them and the tent collapses. For example, if there are patients but not a motivated staff, you can be sure to have a fruitless practice. And the converse: if there is a motivated staff but no patients, you can be sure of the same disappointing results.

After reading this article, you will have dozens of marketing ideas that can be implemented inexpensively and that can be used immediately, leading to happier patients, a more enthusiastic staff, and greater enjoyment for urologists and their urologic practices.

Marketing to the patients already in a practice

In years past, urologists relied on word of mouth or relationships established during medical training as they opened an office and built their medical practices. Today, however, having a successful practice often requires using marketing principles targeted toward existing patients. Yes, it is nice to get new patients, but it is more

E-mail address: neilb89@aol.com

0094-0143/05/$ - see front matter © 2005 Elsevier Inc. All rights reserved.
doi:10.1016/j.ucl.2005.04.003

important to keep the existing ones. In most businesses, keeping a customer costs one fifth of what it costs to acquire a new one [1]; urology practices are no exception to this rule. If practices are not doing a good job with existing patients, then spending thousands of dollars on a marketing plan to bring in new patients turns no profit. The patients they have right now are the backbone of their practice. Focus on giving these patients the proper care they deserve.

Give your practice a checkup

Listening to patients' impressions of a practice improves the quality of the care they receive. Look at a practice from the patients' perspective. An even better method is to ask patients what they think.

Four effective techniques for determining how patients perceive a practice and for evaluating performance and reputation are

1. Creating a focus group
2. Using a suggestion box
3. Commissioning a "mystery shopper" evaluation
4. Conducting written and oral patient surveys

By seeking feedback, through all or just one of these four methods, practices gain profitable information. Written patient surveys probably are the most popular method of obtaining feedback from patients. Written surveys can be given to patients at the time of their office visits or sent in the mail. The advantages of sending a survey are allowing patients to remain anonymous and to complete the survey at their leisure. The

disadvantages are that this is more expensive and people often do not return them.

The easiest, least expensive, and most useful way to survey existing patients is to provide them with a brief questionnaire at every visit. When the patient checks in with the receptionist, they are given a card (Fig. 1) and asked to complete it when they are taken to the examination room. Because this brief questionnaire has yes and no answers, it is easy to tabulate by simply counting the number of yes and no answers. Also, any comments, positive or negative, are answered each day by someone in the office. Such a simple survey is an effective method to take the pulse of a practice and also to hear about the needs and wants of existing patients. These survey comments are a gold mine. Just address the concerns and you will be a hit with existing patients who will remain loyal to the practice and who can help promote the practice to other patients.

Don't be late for a very important date

Ask any patient what he or she dislikes about the health care experience and nearly everyone mentions, "waiting for the doctor." Spending time in waiting rooms probably accounts for more patient dissatisfaction than any other aspect of medical care. One patient puts it this way: "Physicians consistently double-book, stacking us up in the waiting room like planes on a runway. At least with the airlines you get a free drink" [2]. All of us can be more sensitive to patients' number-one complaint: doctors do not respect patients' time. In today's fast-paced, consumer-oriented society, patients expect to be seen and treated promptly. Waiting for the doctor for 30 to 60 minutes or

---

Thank you for helping us to serve you better!

1. Was it easy for you to get an appointment in this office?
   ___ Yes   ___ No
2. Is your general impression of this office favorable?
   ___ Yes   ___ No
3. Was the office staff friendly and concerned?
   ___ Yes   ___ No
4. Did the doctor adequately answer your questions?
   ___ Yes   ___ No
5. Would you recommend this office to someone else?
   ___ Yes   ___ No
6. Do you have any additional comments?

Neil Baum, M.D.
UROLOGY

What three questions would you like answered today?

1. _____
   _____
2. _____
   _____
3. _____
   _____

Please complete the back of this card.

Fig. 1. Patient questionnaire.

more may have been tolerated years ago, but it no longer is acceptable to most patients today.

Patients understand and appreciate good customer service. It goes without saying that good service is prompt service. Keeping patients waiting for excessive periods without explanation sends a message that the doctor's time is more valuable than theirs. Patients interpret this abuse of their time as discourteous and disrespectful. Avoid this impression of your practice at all costs. So, where to start?

Conduct a time and motion study for several weeks. This gives hard facts about how time is managed in a practice. To conduct the study, attach a time and motion sheet (Box 1) to the front of each patient's chart. Record the time the patient arrives, the time of the scheduled appointment, the time the patient was seen, and the time the patient leaves the office. This technique identifies problem areas and offers potential solutions to such problems.

After patients are surveyed and a time and motion study conducted, examine office scheduling procedures. Do staff members double book in an effort to finish the day early? Do they fail to triage patients adequately and allow nonemergency situations to create excessive waits for patients who have scheduled appointments? Review these questions at staff meetings to identify strengths and weaknesses. Look for specific examples of scheduling problems and discuss them with staff. After conducting a time and motion study in my practice, I found that we started falling behind and were experiencing delays at about 2:30 to 3:00 each afternoon. This is when there were one or two urgencies and emergencies that had to be seen and were told to come to the office and they would be worked in. As a result the scheduled patients at the end of the day were delayed 30 to 45 minutes. Solution? After conducting the time and motion study, we created a 20-minute "sacred" time segment each afternoon from 2:50 to 3:10. We leave this segment open during afternoon office hours to accommodate add-ons and emergencies. We do not fill that 20-minute slot for that day until the office opens in the morning. As a result, there is no worry about this time being used for patient care. This 20-minute segment almost always gets used, if not with seeing patients, then with catching up on dictation and patient callbacks. The time and motion study made my practice more sensitive to the patients' time and made my practice more user friendly for the patients.

Finally, encourage staff to develop an on-time mentality. Empower staff to move you along if patients are waiting or appear to be anxious. What works for me is seeing the time and motion sheet on a patient's chart. There may be other signals that help you move along, such as a certain piece of music (eg, Ravel's *Bolero*) or another audible cue that you and your staff agree on. My staff has created humorous cards printed with "Hustle Your Bustle" and "Let's Move It" that are flashed in front of me when I begin running behind schedule.

The bottom line: in many ways, effective time management boils down to plain good manners and practice of the golden rule: If patients are treated the way you like to be treated, chances are good that they will continue to be loyal to you and your practice. Today, being on time is vital to retaining patients. Also, encourage new patients to enter a practice by developing a reputation in the community of being an on-time doctor.

Calling key patients

The best way to keep existing patients in a practice is to call key patients at home. By incorporating this technique into a daily routine,

---

Box 1. Time and motion sheet

Patient name _____
Date _____
_____Scheduled appointment
_____Patient arrival time
_____Time patient was brought into examination room
_____Time physicians spent with patient (minutes)
_____Time patient left office
_____Total time in office/time with doctor

you can save time and endear yourself to existing patients. Key patients are those for whom you need to go that extra mile. Key patients often need extra reassurance or follow-up. Here are examples of key patients I have identified in my practice:

Patients seen for outpatient procedures

If I do an outpatient circumcision or hydrocelectomy, I call the patient at home after the sedation has worn off. Calling patients at this time improves their understanding of the findings and recommendations significantly.

Patients recently discharged from the hospital

These patients usually have questions regarding medications, allowed activities, and follow-up appointments. Even the most careful discharge planning by hospital nurses does not answer all their questions.

Patients sent for diagnostic studies (for example, a CT scan to differentiate cyst from tumor)

These patients do not want to wait until their next appointment for the results. Certainly, if the tests are positive or suggest a hospital admission or surgery, you may want to discuss these results with the patient in person.

Patients who in the past would have been admitted to the hospital but today are managed as outpatients

Examples are patients who have epididymitis or acute pyelonepritis and patients seen for urinary retention who are sent home with a Foley catheter. They always appreciate being called at home and feel reassured that you are concerned about their health and well-being.

Patients new to a practice

Simply call these patients and say, "I just want you to know it was really nice to meet you in the office. I want to make sure that I've answered all your questions."

Ideally, you should be the one to call the key patients, but this is not always possible. If you are unable to contact a key patient, have the nurse make the call. Nurses can triage patients' questions and inform you if they have any questions that they cannot answer.

The bottom line on calling key patients: the best way to promote a practice is to contact key patients at home. Give it a try; you will not be disappointed. Calling key patients could be the key to unlocking marketing success.

Attracting new patients to a practice

The backbone of attracting new patients to a practice is to become visible within the community. There are few urologists who have the luxury of simply hanging out a shingle and waiting for the patients to knock the door down. Most have to make a definite, planned strategy to let the public know who they are, where they practice, and what their areas of interest and expertise are. This enables them to build practices and to attract new patients. Marketing is just one element that allows them to accomplish this goal. Of course, they still have to be cost effective, demonstrate excellent outcomes, and provide outstanding service, but first, get the patients to call the office for an appointment. There is no shortcut to accomplishing this goal or objective. Become a public speaker and writer for local magazines and newspapers, get attention from radio and TV media, and, finally, make use of the internet.

Internet marketing

Tens of millions of patients use the internet to get health care information, and, according to a recent *Wall Street Journal* survey, more than half of patients are making connections to the internet as a direct result of a visit to their physician. A recent report by Cyber Dialogue estimates that more than 33 million patients are willing to switch to physicians who have practice Web sites and offer e-mail access to their practice.

Having an internet presence means more than taking an office brochure and putting it on the World Wide Web. Patients are looking for real value from Web pages and brochure-ware does not make a page attractive or, in the language of the internet, will not make the Web site "sticky"—making people stay on the page, read the content, and, more importantly, contact the office for an appointment. Today, Web surfers and consumers are looking for interactive approaches that make their overall experiences specific, unique, and customized. Sites must offer outstanding clinical content that is credentialed by legitimate medical sources, such as medical societies (eg, www.afud.org, www.auanet.org, or www.ama-assn.org), and offer practices office tools, such as secure messaging, appointment scheduling, insurance verification, prescription refills, and other applications that can make the running of a medical office more streamlined and efficient.

Many internet-savvy consumers are seeking information on specific urologic procedures, such as vasectomy and vasectomy reversal. Indeed, there are approximately 500,000 vasectomies performed in the United States annually and an estimated 50,000 reversals.

How to connect with this growing, high-quality patient base that basically knows what it wants, is decision ready, offers excellent potential for patient retention, and usually is ready to pay for their procedures?

General physician database listings may generate more exposure for physician practices. These listings, however, are not procedure specific. As a result, patients must jump or surf from other information resources to databases to find what they are seeking. In addition, physicians who are contacted through general physician database listings have no way of knowing if patients are financially prepared for elective-service procedures, such as vasectomy reversal.

There are internet sites that can help connect patients with procedure-specific information. In urology, one site that provides comprehensive information on vasectomy and vasectomy reversal, along with a user-friendly physician database, is www.vasectomy.com.

Established in 1999, www.vasectomy.com is an alliance of physicians that differs in many respects from many other medical sites. This site provides potential patients with a resource that supplements the information that they receive before their first office visit. This Web site originally was intended to provide basic consumer information. Now the site is the only online resource from doctors performing these procedures and offers all of the following at one internet location:

- Authoritative information: nearly 100 information-rich pages, including feature and secondary articles illustrations, reference charts, and other resources that provide authoritative information based on the most common questions and issues expressed by patients and site visitors.
- Physician database: free access to physician practices that professionally showcase physicians and practices in a highly credible editorial environment. Each participating doctor can upgrade to a personal biography page for prospective local patients. These are interactive pages that allow patients to request an appointment online, link to practices' Web sites, and produce a map to the offices. In addition, new patient forms can be downloaded by patients and completed at home, thereby saving office staff time in preparing forms to be sent out and reducing patient time in the office filling out those forms.
- Affordability options: when cost remains a concern, www.vasectomy.com suggests affordability options for patients to consider. These include paying in cash (sometimes earning a discount), the use of major credit cards, medical financing agencies, or a combination of options. It is good business for practices to help bring a desired procedure within financial reach of a patient family.

Also, do not forget that marketing a Web site means informing current patients of the existence of the Web page. Simple suggestions include placing the Web address on letterhead and business cards, placing notices in the reception (not waiting) area and examination rooms, and adding Web addresses to office yellow page listings.

A marketing pearl to attract new patients: provide easy access to the practice—make every effort to see that patients can contact their physicians by telephone or by e-mail and that patients do not have to wait for a long time to make an appointment. This applies especially to new patients. New patients who have a urologic problem do not want to wait for 4 to 6 weeks to get an appointment with a doctor.

Bottom line: patients are demanding online access to physician offices, and those doctors who do not take notice of the importance of the internet have the potential to lose online patients. Using the internet to market practices can result in an increase in revenue, reduced expenses, improved efficiency, and improvement in the quality of care offered to patients.

Motivating staff to market and promote practices

The greatest surgical skills and the greatest marketing program all may be wasted if staff does not place a priority on satisfying the needs and the wants of the patients. All the marketing efforts can be ruined if a receptionist places a patient on hold for several minutes or a staff member is rude to a patient or family member. Try a few of these nonmonetary methods to help motivate staff and thereby ensure that every patient has a stellar experience with you and your practice:

1. Perform a fair performance review. I believe employees like to know where they stand and

how they can improve performance on the job. Motivated staff members want feedback on their progress—or even lack of progress. I suggest meeting with employees on a scheduled basis, approximately every 3 to 4 months. At that time, constructively review their performance. I give each employee a worksheet (Box 2) before the scheduled review.

2. Encourage continuing education. Motivating staff often requires outside assistance and training. I believe it is a good investment to encourage employees to participate in various continuing education courses and support their efforts financially.

3. Empower staff. Most urologists have learned to delegate the responsibility of running the office. The most successful urologists have learned to empower employees to take control and assume responsibility for their decisions and actions.

    In my office, employees who have been with the practice 6 months to 1 year can make financial decisions up to $200 without consulting me. When employees are given the freedom to make responsible decisions, you let them know that you care about them.

4. Promote a positive mental attitude. A positive mental attitude can be promoted by surrounding employees with motivational statements, such as, "It is not your aptitude but your attitude that determines your altitude." Another is to provide employees with golden attitude pins to be worn on their uniforms. These pins serve as reminders that every employee is expected to enter the office each day with a golden attitude.

5. Recognize achievement. Nothing is more motivating for employees than for physicians to recognize their achievements and accomplishments. When you recognize improvement in job performance, tell the person directly. You are satisfying that employee's need for self-esteem. This improves employees' confidence and also helps them fulfill the need for self-esteem from fellow employees.

6. Use distinctive uniforms. I think it is important for staff morale for the office uniforms to be different from the customary white ones. Make your uniforms distinctive and people remember you for your signature colors.

7. Show staff you care. Employees need to know that you care about them not just as workers but also as individuals with their own personal lives. When my employees or their family members are sick, I call them at home to check on them and make sure that they have access to adequate medical care.

8. Catch staff doing things right. I am a real believer in the idea that praise and compliments are much appreciated. I send specific thank-you notes acknowledging employees going the extra mile and making an extra effort on behalf of patients. I have two other ways to thank employees who go the extra mile and exceed patients' expectations of our practice. One is the extra mile-o-gram (Fig. 2) and the other is a thanks-a-million check (Fig. 3).

9. Reward staff for saving money or reducing expenses. If a staff member comes up with an idea that saves the practice money, give a bonus. I am trying to motivate my staff

---

Box 2. Performance review questionnaire

1. What do you like most about working here? _____

2. What one or two things would you recommend to improve?
   Working conditions_____
   Morale_____
   Teamwork_____

3. Where do you want to be professionally
   Next quarter?_____
   Six months from now?_____
   One year from now?_____

4. What can I do to help you reach your goals?_____

5. What are you going to do to reach your goals?_____

6. Any other comments or suggestions:_____

not just to earn more money for the practice but also to reduce expenses. They are paid for identifying and designing money-saving ideas.

11. Surprise is the spice of life. Whenever you can provide an unexpected perk for staff, you can be sure that they will appreciate the gesture. In one instance, one employee was on vacation and another employee was ill at home. We all had to work harder to take up the slack for 5 days. In spite of being shorthanded, we were able to function at regular speed and capacity without affecting the quality of care provided for our patients. Our extra effort was so successful that our patients were not even aware of the shortfall that was taking place in our office! I was so impressed with the extra effort that I arranged for a massage therapist to visit our practice on Friday afternoon and give

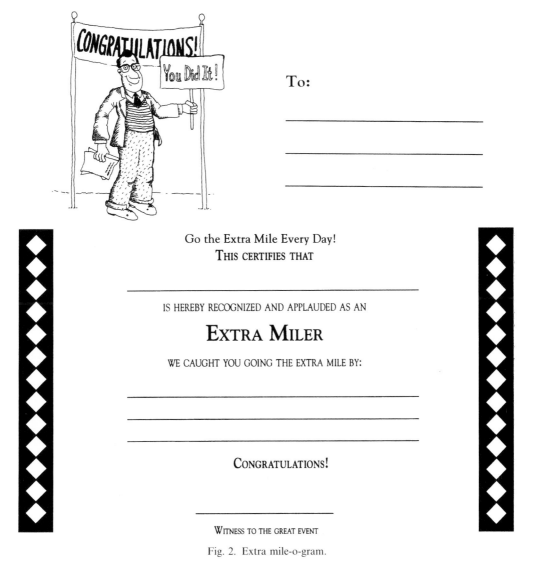

Fig. 2. Extra mile-o-gram.

everyone a 15- to 20-minute massage as a way of saying thank you.

The bottom line on staff motivation: encouraging staff to develop team spirit makes good business sense. When employees have a personal investment in problem solving and decision making, they go the extra mile for the patients and the practice. And remember, properly rewarding employees can be accomplished with minimal expense, energy, and effort.

Improving communications with referral sources

The fourth pillar of the marketing plan for urologists is marketing to other physicians. Whether or not you have a solo private practice or are a partner of a large multispecialty practice, marketing to colleagues should be at the top of your list. The key to physician marketing is to find ways to make their professional lives easier when they deal with you and your practice.

The most essential element of a total marketing plan is to make a practice user friendly. Nowhere is this more important than in the area of working with referring physicians.

The main strategy for getting physician referrals is to have your name cross the minds and desks of referring physicians and their staff members frequently and in a positive fashion. If you can do that, physician referrals will come your way. There should be good chemistry between you and your referring physicians. If they have good feelings about you, they will want to refer patients to you. Make yourself more attractive to referring physicians by making it easy to do business or work with you and your staff.

When referring physicians are surveyed about why they make referrals, they list the following in order of preference:

- Prompt reporting
- Teaching
- Gifts and entertaining

Always keep your physicians informed about their patients' progress. When you see patients by referral, follow this cardinal rule: never allow patients to arrive back in the referring physicians' office before your report arrives on the physician's desk. If you are looking for the best way to make yourself accessible to your referring physicians, consider prompt reporting. Nothing is more embarrassing to referring physicians than to be in the dark about what is going on with a patient. If a patients calls her gynecologist to talk about estrogen replacement therapy and emaciation to treat her incontinence and that doctor has not received your report, you not only look bad in the eyes of the gynecologist but also the efficiency of your practice grinds to a halt. Now your staff has to retrieve the patient's chart, and you are interrupted to answer any questions that the gynecologist may have.

The usual communication between a specialist and the referring doctor is 7 to 10 days after a patient is seen. During that hiatus, the patient often beats the letter back to the referring doctor. A technique for handling this is to use the "lazy

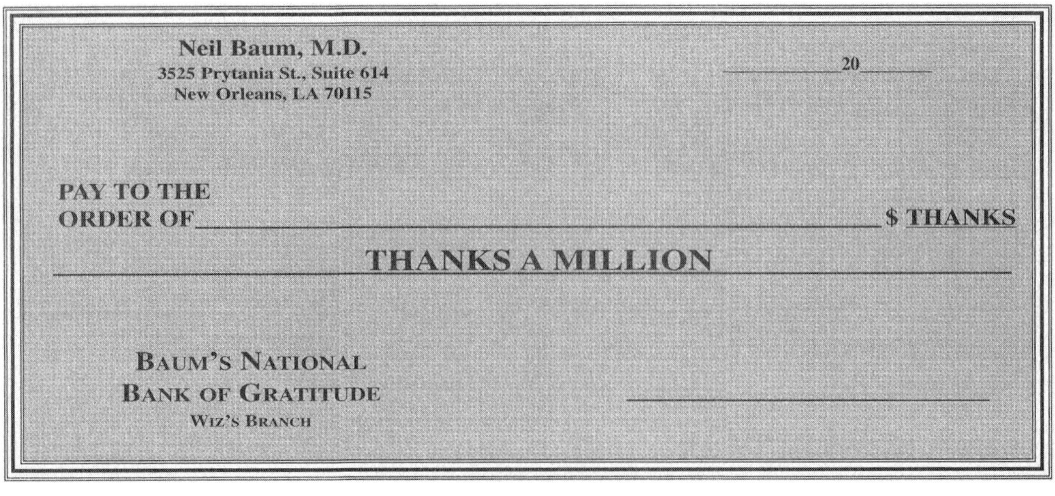

Neil Baum, M.D.
3525 Prytania St., Suite 614
New Orleans, LA 70115

_____ 20 _____

PAY TO THE
ORDER OF_____ $ THANKS

_____ THANKS A MILLION _____

BAUM'S NATIONAL
BANK OF GRATITUDE
WIZ'S BRANCH

_____

Fig. 3. Thanks a million check.

person's referral letter." This requires no dictating and guarantees that 100% of the time, the letter beats the patient back to the referring doctor. The three most important aspects of the referral letter are the diagnosis, the medications, and the treatment plan. These ingredients are referred to as the buzz words. These words are circled in the progress notes of the chart. For instance, a man is seen with a problem of mild to moderate benign prostatic hyperplasia and you recommend a trial of α-blockers. You plan to see him back in the office and check on his progress in 2 months. These key words are circled in the chart. At the end of the day, the nurse goes through the chart after the patient's visit and looks for the key words you have circled. She calls up a boilerplate referral letter on the computer screen, which has blanks for completion (Box 3). The nurse types in the appropriate referring physician's name, the diagnosis, and so forth. The letter is printed and faxed directly to the physician's office the same afternoon that the patient is seen.

This type of referral letter delivers the essentials to referring physicians immediately. Whenever referring physicians receive a two- to three-page dictated report, they look first for the diagnosis, recommended treatment plan, and the follow-up recommendations. Referring doctors simply do not have time to read a long report.

If patients call a referring doctor with any questions, then they can answer them without having to contact you or your office for clarification. Furthermore, the letter usually can be generated without any dictating at all. If you survey referring doctors, most indicate that they prefer a timely computerized referral letter to a delayed three-pager. Some specialists are concerned that referring physicians are upset when they receive a computerized, impersonal form letter, but surveys of referring physicians indicate that they value timely information more than a delayed personal letter.

There are other economic considerations involved in using the lazy person's referral letter. The typical referral letter can cost anywhere from $13.50 to $25.00 or more every time you pick up the tape recorder. Using the lazy person's referral letter reduces costs to under $1 per letter. Plus, it satisfies the needs and wants of primary care physicians—the letters arrive before patients return.

One method of keeping primary care physicians informed is to send a do-it-yourself newsletter about the latest developments in your specialty. After attending a conference, you have more than enough information for a short, one-page newsletter that educates referring physicians about the latest developments.

Also, make an effort to recognize referring physicians' accomplishments and those of their children. There is no better way to enhance your relationship with referring physicians than to acknowledge their accomplishments. It is a friendly gesture to cut out articles from local newspapers that mention referring physicians or their families. Whenever referring physicians receive an appointment or promotion, acknowledge it with a written note.

Finally, keep referring physicians abreast of changes in your specialty. Approximately once or twice a year, after I attend a meeting of urologists, I send out a single-sheet informal newsletter about the latest developments in my practice and in urology in general. These newsletters often are much appreciated by referring physicians. Samples of those newsletters are available on the internet at www.urologychannel.com/neilbaum.

Intraspecialty referrals

You also can develop referrals from urology colleagues. Just because you are a urologist does not mean you cannot get referrals from other urologists. You may be doing procedures or

---

Box 3. Boilerplate lazy person's referral letter

Dear [Referring Physician],
[Patient]_____ was seen for a problem of [diagnosis], and he/she is being treated
with [medications] _____. I recommend that he/she have [treatment
plan] _____. I will see him/her again in [time to next visit] and
I will keep in touch with you regarding her/her urologic progress.
Sincerely,
Neil Baum, MD

diagnostic tests that they are not doing and that may be helpful to them. You may have equipment or training they do not have, enabling you to develop referrals from colleagues in your specialty.

Let colleagues know that you are willing to see their patients and give their patients back. The easiest way to do this and make your colleagues feel secure is to offer to help at their institutions. See a referred patient in your office, but admit the patient to a colleague's hospital and get temporary privileges at that hospital. In that way, the referring physician gets to see the procedure and has the security of knowing you are not taking the patient away.

Nontraditional referrals

Urologists have the opportunity to communicate with other health care professionals who could be sources of referrals. Health care professionals, such as nurses, hospital employees, pharmacists, and pharmaceutical representatives, are frequently asked by family and friends to make recommendations for a urologist. For example, nurses and hospital employees frequently are asked whom they should see for urologic problems. Giving talks to the nurses at your hospital and in the community can serve as an excellent method of letting these professionals know about your area of interest in management of specific urologic problems.

Pharmacists are another group from whom patients frequently seek advice. It is important to become any ally of the pharmacists in the community. Pharmaceutical representatives and medical manufacturing representatives also are resources, not only for generating good public relations but also for serving as referral sources for your practice. If pharmaceutical representatives see that you have an area of interest in a special urologic area, they will recommend your practice to other physicians, friends, and family. If you want to endear yourself to the drug representatives and other sales people who call on your practice, see them in a timely fashion. That is their "hot button," and they appreciate that you do not ignore them or keep them waiting.

One way to improve the efficiency of time spent with pharmaceutical representatives is to request an agenda letter. This letter asks them to inform you on the nature and length of time they expect to spend to discuss their product or drug. You then can decide if you want to see the representative about that subject and can indicate that you accept their time frame. This method focuses the representative's visit significantly and reduces the amount of time that spent with them to obtain information on their products.

The bottom line: marketing yourself to colleagues does not mean that you are trying to take away market share. When you open up possibilities, you actually increase their business and yours. The way in which you do this does not take away; it just adds to your stature in the professional community, to the respect you get from your peers, and to the bottom line.

Summary

In this new millennium, success will not belong to urologists who have merely the newest piece of technology for treating benign prostatic hyperplasia in the office setting or to physicians who simply purchase the largest advertisements in the yellow pages. Success will belong to those urologists who practice good quality medicine and put a premium on giving the best possible service.

Marketing is not a 1-day, 1-week, or 1-year commitment; it is lifelong. To have the desired successful practice, you always will be marketing and promoting services. Always search for ways to satisfy patients, staff, colleagues, and payers. Make an effort to exceed their expectations about their experience with you and your practice. Try incremental improvements, pay attention to the details, as they really do make a big difference, and reevaluate continually to see what works and what does not—for you and for those who come in contact with the practice.

Remember,

> When a person or practice fails,
> Some people call it fate.
> More often it is bad marketing
> Discovered far too late.

References

[1] Sellers P. Getting customers to love you. Fortune March 3, 1989. p. 38–9.
[2] USA Today. August 15, 1999.

ELSEVIER
SAUNDERS

Urol Clin N Am 32 (2005) 309–317

UROLOGIC
CLINICS
of North America

Retirement Plans for Physicians and Their Employees

Joel M. Blau, CFP™

MEDIQUS Asset Advisors, Inc., 200 North LaSalle Street, Chicago, IL 60601, USA

In the past, urologists planned for retirement by reviewing a potentially expansive list of income sources, such as social security, pensions from health care organizations, and income from investment portfolios. Today, planning for retirement is more focused on areas that physicians are able to control and to which they can contribute. For example, now it is appropriate to question whether or not social security will be available for retirement income. It is becoming more important to plan well in advance for the income needs that will exist during retirement.

One of the greatest benefits of any business is the ability to contribute on a tax-deductible basis to retirement plans. When businesses are a medical practices, the owners choose a plan that can benefit their personal situation best and create long-term incentives for their employees.

As more urologists become aware of their own need to plan for retirement income security, qualified retirement plans remain the logical starting point. Qualified retirement plans generally are classified as defined benefit or defined contribution. Some plans combine features of both types.

Defined-benefit plans

Defined-benefit plans tend to favor older, highly compensated employees, such as physicians who are close to retirement. That is because employers have fewer years over which to accumulate enough money to provide a promised benefit. Actuarial calculations are made to determine how much money must be contributed each year to accumulate the necessary future amount. Interest rates, investment rates of return, and ages of participants have an impact on calculations. Investment risks

rest solely on employers, who are required to fund the plan adequately each year, although the annual contribution can vary based on a plan's investment results. The future benefit received may be based on a flat percentage of compensation, a percentage that increases with length of service, a percentage that changes at certain compensation levels, or several other formulas.

There are many advantages to the employees. First, these plans are funded completely by employers, and neither contributions nor earnings are taxed to employees when they are in these plans. Also, employees have peace of mind knowing they receive a future benefit. Many plans even allow employees to borrow from the plan within certain strict guidelines.

The primary disadvantage of defined-benefit plans relates to younger plan participants. Younger employees generally receive a smaller portion of the total contribution, primarily because of the longer time period before their retirement. From an employer's standpoint, some advantages of defined-benefit plans are:

- The ability to reward long-term employees with a substantial retirement benefit even though they are close to retirement age.
- Forfeitures from terminating employees reduce future funding requirements for current employees.
- Plan investments are directed solely by employers.

Although once the qualified retirement plan of choice for many medical practices, defined-benefit plans have become less popular because of the following disadvantages to employers:

- In low-profit years, employers still are obligated to make plan contributions.
- Investment risks rest solely with employers.

E-mail address: blau@mediqus.com

0094-0143/05/$ - see front matter © 2005 Elsevier Inc. All rights reserved.
doi:10.1016/j.ucl.2005.03.006

- Administration costs are higher than for defined-contribution plans, because an actuary must be retained to certify the reasonableness of contributions and deductions.

Recent legislation, however, has lifted other defined-benefit obstacles, and its popularity is on the rise again. Defined-benefit plans afford significant contribution and deduction opportunities.

Defined-contribution plans

There are several variations of defined-contribution plans commonly used by medical practices: money purchase pension plans, profit-sharing plans, age-weighted profit-sharing plans, new comparability plans, 401(k) savings plans, and savings incentive match plans for employees (SIMPLEs).

Money purchase pension plans

In money purchase pension plans, employers contribute a specified percentage of the total participating employees' salaries each year. This contribution is allocated among the participants. Up to 25% of a participant's payroll can be contributed and deducted by employers. Plan contributions can be based on total compensation, including bonuses and overtime pay. Maximum recognized compensation for 2005 is $210,000, which is indexed for inflation in future years. A participant's annual account contribution may not exceed which is less: 100% of compensation or $42,000 per year.

Money purchase pension plans typically favor younger participants because they have a longer time period over which their accounts grow. In many instances, they share in plan forfeitures. Forfeitures occur when participants leave a practice before they are 100% vested. The nonvested forfeitures then are reallocated to the remaining participants, thus benefiting employees who remain in the plan the longest.

In addition to the deductibility of contributions, there are other advantages for employers:

- Contributions and administrative costs are known in advance.
- Contributions rise as compensation rises, but they are controllable by formula and absolute dollar amounts.
- Employers can direct the investment portfolio, or employees can self-direct their own portions of the plan.

The primary disadvantage to employers stems from mandatory contributions. Employers are obligated to make contributions, even in years when practices lose money. The primary disadvantage to employees is the lack of a guarantee of the amount of retirement benefit, because the investment risks rest on employee participants, regardless of who directs the investments. Money purchase pension plans are all but extinct. Profit-sharing plans allow for up to the same 25% of salary contributions, but on a year-by-year discretionary basis.

Profit-sharing plans

For greater employer flexibility, profit-sharing plans may be the defined-contribution plan of choice. Employer contributions to these plans need not be made every year. The maximum annual deduction is limited to 25% of compensation, with an individual recognized maximum compensation of $210,000 (as of January 1, 2005).

Although annual contributions generally are discretionary, if there are profits, employers are expected to make substantial and recurring contributions. As a rule of thumb, contributions in 3 out of 5 years or 5 out of 10 years usually satisfy the Internal Revenue Service (IRS).

For employees, profit-sharing plans tend to favor younger participants. The down sides of profit-sharing plans, however, are similar to those of money purchase pension plans. There are no guarantees of the amount of future retirement benefits, and investment risks rest on employees. In addition, there is no assurance of the frequency and amount of employer contributions. Advantages of profit-sharing plans to employers include:

- Providing incentive to employees to be productive to maximize the profit potential of the practice
- Contributions that are totally flexible
- Forfeitures of terminating employees are reallocated among active participants, generally with a greater percentage allocated to the highest salaried participants, such as the physicians

Although contribution limits of profit-sharing plans are set at 25% of covered payroll, this type of plan generally does not produce contributions and deductions for older employees that are as large as those with defined-benefit plans.

Age-weighted profit-sharing plans

Because defined-contribution plans tend to favor younger employees, an alternative is age-weighted profit-sharing plans. Employer contributions in this type of plan are not necessarily based on profits. Contributions are totally flexible and at the discretion of employers. Contributions need not be made yearly, as long as they are substantial and recurring. Employer contributions are allocated to provide an equal retirement benefit at normal retirement age for all participants. Older participants are favored from a contribution perspective because they are closer to retirement. All participants, however, receive the same projected retirement benefit percentage at age 65. Age-weighted profit-sharing plans do have potential disadvantages for employers:

- If the key employees are younger than other employees, they do not receive as large a proportion of employer contributions.
- Administrative costs are higher because of actuarial calculations.
- It is more difficult to explain these plans to employees.

New comparability plans

As if the scope of retirement plan alternatives is not complex enough, recent IRS regulations allow businesses and professional practices to establish a hybrid profit-sharing plan, known as new comparability plans. These plans allow for substantial contributions to be made to a favored and, on average, older group, with much lower contributions for other employees. In certain situations, annual contributions for tax year 2005 can be as high as 100% of income, up to a maximum of $42,000, for each member of a highly compensated group of employees, such as physicians, and as low as 5% of pay for younger non–highly compensated employees.

This new allocation method is made possible by IRS regulations, which allow employers to divide plan participants into one or more classes and, in many cases, make larger contributions for one class than for another. Section 401(a)(4) of the IRS code states as a requirement for plan qualification that "contributions *or* benefits provided under the plan do not discriminate in favor of highly compensated employees". The justification for the new comparability plan lies in the word "or" and is based on an analysis of projected benefits at retirement age, showing that the benefits provided to highly compensated and non–highly compensated employees are comparable and, therefore, considered nondiscriminatory. This is the same justification behind the popular and widely used age-weighted profit-sharing plans, which provide a greater benefit for older employees.

With new comparability plans, the percentage of a plan's contribution going to the owners, partners, or highly compensated employees (such as urologists who are not partners) in a practice can be higher than with traditional age-weighted profit-sharing plans. This is because, unlike age-based or -weighted plans, new comparability plans allow participants to be divided into classes, with one favored older class (highly compensated employees) receiving a much higher level of contribution than the other class (all of the non–highly compensated employees). New comparability plans generally are ideal for practices that have owners or partners who

- Are older, on average, than their other employees.
- Want the contribution flexibility of profit-sharing plans versus the mandatory contributions of defined-benefit pension plans.
- Want the largest share of the plan contribution allocated to their own accounts.

401(k) plans

Urologists no longer can be content maximizing retirement plan contributions and assuming they will have sufficient assets to create a comfortable retirement standard of living. The stock markets over the years have taken many prisoners, as evidenced by investors who jumped on the high-growth technology bandwagon in the late 1990s only to find that their portfolios declined in value by more than 50% during the successive 3-years bear market cycle. This situation was a reminder for many physicians approaching retirement age to reevaluate their options, to determine if they will be forced to work longer or work at a reduced level during retirement.

Younger urologists also felt the impact, as portfolio rates of return fell well below their initial expectations. Although the market will continue to move in various cycles, negatively and positively, now is the time for urologists to reevaluate their qualified retirement plans to be certain they are taking advantage of the new increased limits and understand the major change affecting 401(k) plans.

IRS code section 401(k) retirement savings programs allow employees to contribute on their own behalf, on a pretax basis, with the benefit of tax-deferred compounding similar to traditional individual retirement accounts (IRAs), pension plans, and profit-sharing plans. The maximum allowable pretax contribution for employees is $14,000 for 2005. Employees who are age 50 and older may be able to contribute an additional $4,000 via the catch-up deferral. In order for physicians to be able to contribute the maximum allowable amount to their 401(k) plans, there also must be participation from the lower compensated employees to ensure that plans are not discriminatory.

A traditional 401(k) plan is subject to two nondiscrimination tests—the actual deferral percentage test for employee elective deferrals and the actual contribution percentage test for matching contributions. As an alternative, employers may adopt a safe harbor 401(k) plan, which is not subject to nondiscrimination testing.

Under current tax law, there are two safe harbor alternatives to the actual deferral percentage test. In the first, employers make a nonelective contribution of 3% to each eligible highly compensated and non–highly compensated employee. The other alternative offers employers an opportunity to make matching contributions of 100% of non–highly compensated employee elective contributions up to 3% of pay and 50% of non–highly compensated employee additional elective contributions up to 5% of pay. All matches and nonelective contributions made to satisfy the safe harbor must be vested immediately. In addition, employers must notify employees within a reasonable period of time, before the plan year, of their rights and obligations under the safe harbor arrangement.

By meeting these criteria, many highly compensated owners and physicians find they actually are able to accrue a greater benefit for themselves. With the objective of most qualified retirement plans being tax advantaged growth for future income needs, the greater amount allowed to be invested annually can make a dramatic difference down the road. Often acting as contribution limitations, guidelines are in place to ensure that there is not a great disparity of contributions, with highly compensated key employees receiving the lion's share. The safe harbor alternative to the traditional 401(k) plan enables many urologists to accrue a greater retirement benefit while conforming to IRS guidelines. Based on the history of prior employee participation, the safe harbor plan may prove a viable alternative for those who want to maximize their retirement planning options.

Not surprisingly, financial independence remains a primary goal for most urologists. Although the desirability of this goal has not changed over the years, the feasibility of attaining it has. Faced with lower incomes and longer hours, physicians will come to rely more heavily on their portfolio returns, especially within qualified retirement plans, to become financially independent. Either as owners or employees, urologists may be able to have some input into investment decisions to fit their long-term personal objectives better.

According to a United States Chamber of Commerce survey, 80% of businesses with fewer than 100 employees offer defined-contribution plans, whereas only 47% sponsor some type of defined-benefit plan funded solely by employers. With the shift toward profit-sharing and 401(k) plans as the primary retirement funding vehicle, it is imperative to take advantage of its design flexibility to maximize benefits.

Savings incentive match plans for employees

The Small Business Job Protection Act of 1996 created a unique retirement plan—SIMPLE. SIMPLE replaces the salary-reduction version of the simplified employee pension. SIMPLE allows small business owners to put aside money easily and inexpensively in tax-deferred accounts for themselves and their employees.

To take advantage of this new form of retirement savings, business entities must have no more than 100 employees and cannot use any other retirement plan in the same year. Also, eligible employees must have earned at least $5,000 in any 2 previous years from the same employer and be likely to do so in the current year.

SIMPLEs are available in two forms: a SIMPLE IRA and a SIMPLE 401(k). SIMPLE IRAs can be set up for each employee for a nominal fee at a bank, mutual fund company, or brokerage firm. SIMPLE 401(k)s are more expensive mainly because of administrative costs.

SIMPLEs allow owners and employees to defer a percentage of their compensation, up to $10,000 a year, indexed for inflation, with a catch-up provision for workers ages 50 and over, allowing an additional $2,000 to be contributed. Owners may contribute to employees' plans either with a matching contribution of 100% of the first 3% of participating workers' annual compensation deferred, up to a maximum of $10,000, or by contributing 2% of compensation up to $4,200 in 2005 for all workers, whether or not they participate in the salary deferral portion of the plan.

Because SIMPLEs are a newer form of retirement plan, many options must be considered before implementation. On the positive side, SIMPLEs require no discrimination testing (which requires a certain relation between the amount of compensation deferred by the group of participants included in the lower level of compensation and those in the higher level of compensation); employees need not participate for business owners to defer up to $10,000 plus the 3% match per year.

Traditional 401(k) plans limit employers' tax deferral by the amount employees put into a plan. In addition, employers have no fiduciary responsibility for employee investments under the SIMPLE arrangement.

Urologists who want to save more for retirement and take a bigger deduction may find the maximum contribution confining. Other qualified plans allow employers to deduct as much as 100% of their salary up to $42,000 per year. Also, because SIMPLE money is fully vested from the beginning, these plans provide little incentive for employee loyalty.

Table 1 summarizes the basic issues in qualified plan alternatives and should assist in understanding the differences among plans.

Which plan may be the right fit?

There are many factors to consider when evaluating different types of retirement plans for a medical practice. Table 2 helps evaluate the benefits of each and narrow the alternatives. Consulting with retirement experts before making a final decision is critical.

Implementing a plan

To determine the feasibility of implementing a new qualified retirement plan for a practice, be sure to analyze a number of testing models that can compare the current plan with alternatives. An accountant or third-party administrator (TPA) can be a valuable resource in exploring qualified retirement plan options. Typically, TPAs do not offer investment advice but focus exclusively on the mechanics of the plans and assist in the analysis of whether or not the plan options can attain the goals and objectives of the practice owners. Because of the environment of constantly changing tax laws, it generally makes sense to reevaluate retirement plan options on an ongoing basis to ensure taking the greatest advantage of today's tax advantaged opportunities.

Many skilled professionals are available to assist with qualified plan implementation. A TPA helps in plan design, participant information, and governmental reporting. The trustees can take responsibility for investing or can hire an investment manager. An actuary is involved when using defined-benefit plans. Many professional financial organizations can act in multiple capacities. For smaller plans, a practice's accountant may perform the duties of plan administration, whereas principal physicians act as trustees and hire investment professionals to construct and invest the portfolio. Whatever group or entity a medical practice chooses to work with, they must be aware of the goals and objectives that the practice has determined to be in its best interest.

Regardless of the type of plan chosen, care must be taken to observe the tax and legal requirements established by the IRS and the Department of Labor. IRS regulations require the filing of the appropriate tax forms for a plan, such as Form 5500, which reports on the assets, contributions, and expenses of a plan. An accountant or TPA usually handles these matters. Department of Labor requirements include the distribution of required information to plan participants, making distributions to former participants in a timely fashion, and other miscellaneous items.

There is a separate item, which falls under the Department of Labor domain: the need to satisfy a variety of requirements regarding the investment of plan assets. To assist plan trustees, a series of requirements are identified in the Employee Retirement Income Security Act (ERISA). These requirements are:

- An investment policy must be established and should be in writing (ERISA sections 402[a][1], 40229[b][1] to [2], and 404[a][1][D]).
- Plan assets must be diversified (ERISA section 404[a][1][c]).
- Investment decisions must be made with the skill and care of a prudent expert (ERISA section 404[a][1][b]).
- Investment performance must be monitored (ERISA section 405[a]).

Table 1
Qualified plans compared

Feature	Defined-benefit plans	Defined-contribution plans			
	All defined-benefit plans	Money purchase pension	Profit-sharing	Age-weighted profit-sharing	SIMPLE
Employer contributions deductible?	Yes	Yes	Yes	Yes	Yes
Employer contributions to participant currently taxable?	No	No	No	No	No
Earnings accumulate with income tax deferred?	Yes	Yes	Yes	Yes	Yes
Maximum annual employer contributions or deductions?	Determined by actuary	100% of compensation	100% of compensation	100% of compensation	100% match up to 3% of compensation or 2% of compensation of all eligible employees
Employer contributions required?	Yes	Yes	No	No	Yes
Employer contributions are allocated?	N/A	1. As a percentage of total covered compensation 2. Integrated with social security	1. As a percentage of total covered compensation 2. Integrated with social security	Based on number of years before participant reaches retirement age	Pro-rata by compensation

Employee contributions required?	No	No	No	No	No
Maximum participant benefits (for defined-benefit plans) or allocations (for defined-contribution plans)?	Lesser of 100% of compensation or $170,000 annually	Lesser of 25% of compensation or $42,000	Lesser of 25% of compensation or $42,000	Lesser of 25% of compensation or $42,000	Lesser of 100% of compensation or $10,000
Investments can be self-directed by participants?	No	Yes	Yes	Yes	Yes
What plan participants are favored by the plan design?	Older, closer to retirement, highly compensated	Highly compensated	Highly compensated	Older, closer to retirement, highly compensated	Younger
What will participants' account value at retirement depend on?	Formula of the plan, which can be calculated based on years before retirement, compensation, years of service	1. The amount of contributions 2. The number of years until retirement 3. Investment return	1. Frequency and amount of contributions 2. Number of years until retirement 3. Investment return	1. Frequency and amount of contributions 2. Number of years until retirement 3. Investment return	1. Frequency and amount of contributions 2. Number of years until retirement 3. Investment return
Who bears investment risk?	Employer	Employee	Employee	Employee	Employee

Source: Mary Jo Stvan, Oakbrook, Illinois: Merit Benefits.

Table 2
Evaluating retirement plans

Plan type	If flexibility needed in making deposits	If the oldest, most highly compensated, or closest to retirement of all participants	If able to afford contributions that exceed 25% of participant compensation
Defined-benefit	May consider carefully	Definitely consider	Definitely consider
Money purchase pension	Do not consider	Consider	No impact
Profit-sharing	Definitely consider	Unlikely to consider	Consider
Age-weighted profit-sharing	Definitely consider	Definitely consider	Consider
SIMPLE	Definitely consider	Unlikely to consider	Unlikely to consider

- Investment expenses must be controlled (ERISA section 404[a]).
- Prohibited transactions must be avoided (ERISA section 404[a] and [b]).

These requirements make it important for qualified plan trustees to have a general understanding of investments. The allocation of a plan's investment portfolio should be based on many criteria, including the age of the participants, the plan's risk parameters, the plan's expected liabilities, and the type of plan used.

Many urologists act as trustee of a defined-contribution plan and take responsibility for managing a portfolio, either on their own or by hiring an investment advisor. In this situation, there is a pooled fund for all employees and each owns a proportionate share. The problem with this scenario is that employees may have investment objectives based on age, risk tolerance, and required return, which may conflict with those of a physician trustee. To eliminate this potential conflict, many plans offer the ability, through self-direction, for employees to manage and make investment decisions for their portion of a plan's assets. Although this strategy may prove beneficial for plan participants who are astute investors, poor returns can have a devastating effect long term. In addition, trustees must adhere to certain rules to be deemed not responsible for poor investment decisions made by employees. Plan sponsors who follow section 404(c) of ERISA avoid liability for investment losses resulting from participants' control of their portion of a plan. Plan sponsors can elect to not follow ERISA 404(c) and retain fiduciary responsibility for plan investments.

If choosing to allow self-direction of investments by using the code, however, ERISA section 404(c) regulations require that certain information about the plans and about investment alternatives be furnished automatically to all participants.

Required disclosures about investments include the following:

1. A list of the investment options and their specific risks and return characteristics
2. Identification of any designated investment managers
3. A description of any potential transaction fees or expenses
4. An explanation of how to give investment instructions
5. A disclosure that the plan is operating under ERISA section 404(c); thus, plan fiduciaries' responsibility is more limited
6. A commitment to adhere to new mandatory rollover rules to be implemented in 2005

If a plan trustee decides to offer self-direction, it makes sense to follow the ERISA code as a means of limiting liability. A nonfiduciary employee of a group participating in a self-directed retirement plan should be sure that the information listed previously is made available.

Four steps for qualified plan distributions

Persons acting as administrators or as agents responsible for a qualified plan (pension, profit-sharing, 401[k], and so forth) need to know the steps required when employees request a distribution. This typically is done when employees retire or terminate employment.

Administrators are required to give participants who are about to receive a distribution a written explanation covering the following four items:

1. Any special tax treatment for lump sum distributions that may be available to participants
2. If employees are under age $59\frac{1}{2}$ the potential 10% IRS penalty for early withdrawals
3. The regular rollover rules

4. The new mandatory withholding rules and the preferred alternative

The IRS has issued a sample text that can be used to satisfy the required explanation.

Avoiding the early retirement penalty

As a general rule, distributions from qualified plans are subject to a 10% penalty tax if they are withdrawn before participants reach age $59\frac{1}{2}$, become disabled, or die. The term, "qualified plan," includes pensions, profit-sharing plans, simplified employee pensions, Keoghs, IRAs, and 403(b) annuities. Additionally, withdrawals are subject to ordinary income taxation. This reduces premature distribution even further.

When the age $59\frac{1}{2}$ rule was enacted, a general assumption was made that a normal minimum retirement age was 60 years of age. But times have changed! Corporate downsizing has forced many to begin retirement in their mid-50s. Many physicians look at health care reform and consider retiring before the magic age of $59\frac{1}{2}$ How can retirement funds be accessed without paying the 10% penalty?

Depending on personal situations and possible needs for the funds, there are several possible exceptions to the penalty rule. If an objective is simply early retirement, the IRS waives the 10% penalty if the distribution is part of a scheduled series of substantially equal payments. There are three different approved methods when calculating distributions:

1. Single or joint life expectancy method—this method spreads payments over the number of years set forth in the IRS tables based on a single life or joint life, which includes a named beneficiary.
2. Amortization method—using this method, payments are similar to the annual amount required to pay off a loan at a reasonable interest rate over life expectancy.
3. Annuity method—this method uses an annuity factor which has been determined from a reasonable mortality table using a given interest rate assumption. Once beginning annual distributions, they must be continued until age $59\frac{1}{2}$ or for 5 years, whichever is later. Under this rule, 55-year-olds may receive fixed annual distributions to age 60. At that time, they can stop the fixed amount and take out as little or as much as needed from the qualified plan at their own discretion (IRC section 72t).

Even though the three methods may seem similar, they yield different required annual distributions. When considering using the Substantially Equal Payments exception, have an accountant determine each method's results to match income needs and avoid additional income taxation.

Summary

There are many options to consider when comparing and ultimately implementing a qualified retirement plan for a medical practice. Although the tax laws are changing and evolving constantly, historically they have been beneficial relative to specific retirement plan funding limitations and deductions. When either implementing a plan or comparing newer retirement plan options available to a current plan, be sure to work with a retirement plan specialist to assist in the complex decision-making process. If structured in the proper manner, retirement plans help attract and retain key employees, at the same time providing substantial tax advantaged savings plans to assist in reaching financial independence goals.

ELSEVIER
SAUNDERS

Urol Clin N Am 32 (2005) 319–326

UROLOGIC
CLINICS
of North America

General and Cystoscopic Procedures

Joseph W. Akornor, MD[a], Joseph W. Segura, MD[a,b],
Ajay Nehra, MD[a,b],*

[a]Department of Urology, Mayo Clinic, Rochester, MN, USA
[b]Department of Urology, Mayo Clinic College of Medicine, Rochester, MN, USA

History

Cystoscopy and endoscopy have become powerful diagnostic and therapeutic instruments in the evaluation of the urinary tract. The first major advance in endoscopy was in the nineteenth century by a young obstetrician, Phillip Bozzini. In 1806, he designed an instrument that was an elongated thin funnel that could be passed into a large orifice [1]. At the time, the instrument was used for inspection the bladder, rectum, vagina, and nasopharynx. Bozzini's lichtleiter (light conductor) was believed to have insufficient illumination, making it dangerous to use, and was also painful to introduce. In 1826, Pierre Segalas applied the lichtleiter principle to a funnel made of highly polished silver to reflect light [1]. In 1853, Antonin J. Desormeaux introduced his version of a cystoscope [1], which used a concave mirror set at 45° with a central hole used to reflect the light into the organ. Desormeaux often is referred to as the father of cystoscopy for several reasons. He was the first to introduce the lichtleiter into a patient; he is believed to be the surgeon who coined the term endoscopy; and he was the first to use an endoscopic instrument for diagnostic and therapeutic purposes.[1]. The major complication of this instrument was burns. A major advance in optics occurred in 1879, when Max Nitze, working with Leiter, developed a lens system that increased the field of vision [2]. Nitze also introduced the use of prisms to angulate the field of vision by various

degrees and invert the image so it appeared upright [2]. Thomas Edison's invention of the incandescent light bulb in 1880 allowed improvements in Nitze's cystoscope design. In 1889, Boisseau du Rocher separated the cystoscope into two components with a large sheath through which he inserted the lens system [1]. This endoscope was large enough to have channels within the sheath, so that catheters could be passed into the bladder or the bladder could be irrigated. In 1996, Joachim Albarran, a French urologist, added to the Nitze cystoscope a direct method for deflecting the catheter [1]. He invented a thumbscrew that controlled a small lid in the cystoscope, which then elevated or depressed the catheter at its tip in the bladder. In 1959, Hopkins invented the rod-lens system, consisting of a tube of glass with thin lenses of air, resulting in greater visual clarity. Compared with pre World War II systems, the Hopkins system provided a total light transmission that was more than 80 times better [1]. This lens system is used in most rigid endoscopes today.

For many years, the inspection and treatment of lower and upper urinary tract pathology depended solely on rigid instruments with solid lens systems, which provided excellent and clear visualization. The rigid nature of the instrument posed a few problems, including causing significant patient discomfort, especially in males, resulting in suboptimal examination or inadvertent urethral trauma [3]; additionally, patients needed to be in lithotomy position to allow for introduction and adequate manipulation of the instrument, which may have been uncomfortable and difficult for some patients. Lastly, the rigid instrument may have been inadequate because of excessive urethral length (due to a semirigid penile

* Corresponding author. Department of Urology, Mayo Clinic College of Medicine, 200 First Street, SW, Rochester, MN 55905.

E-mail address: nehra.ajay@mayo.edu (A. Nehra).

0094-0143/05/$ - see front matter © 2005 Elsevier Inc. All rights reserved.
doi:10.1016/j.ucl.2005.04.002

urologic.theclinics.com

prosthesis) or lack of urethral compliance (as a result of prior surgery, radiation, or trauma).

To overcome these drawbacks, innovators began to think of ways to navigate anatomic curves using endoscopes. Fiberoptic technology developed rapidly in the 1960s and 1970s, and this led to the development of flexible endoscopes. The earliest reported use of flexible endoscope for examination of bladder neck was by Tsuchida and Sugawara [4]. Since these early reports, flexible cystoscopy has become a universal and integral part of the practice of urology. Flexible cytoscopy provides several advantages over rigid cystoscopy. Flexible cystoscopy provides an excellent diagnostic view of the bladder; patients tolerate the procedure with minimal discomfort; and the entire bladder can be visualized in a few minutes. The procedure can be performed in almost any position, including dorsal lithotomy, supine, and even prone [4]. Patients who have semirigid penile prothesis can be examined easily because of the increased length and maneuverability of the flexible cystoscope [4].

Characteristics of flexible cystoscopes

The basic components of a flexible cystoscope are fiberoptic light-bearing bundles, a single fiberoptic image-bearing bundle, an irrigation working channel, and an active two-way distal tip deflecting mechanism. Several brands of flexible cystoscopes are available (Table 1) with similar features.

The optical system consists of a single image bundle (guide) of coated parallel (coherent) optical fibers that can transmit light when bent, with a guide aligned and fitted to a lens system that magnifies and focuses the image. Because of the coating of each fiber, there is a small space between the fibers in the image guide, thus images appear somewhat granular. The optical system also contains a field marker (a black triangle or outpouching in the visual field) at the 12-o'clock position to help orient the physician during cystoscopy. Light is transmitted by delicate non-coherent fiberoptic bundles that can be damaged by rough handling, perforation of the working channel, or excessive exposure to radiation. Damage to fibers results in either a loss of transmitted light or diminished image. Each broken image fiber results in a representative black dot in the visual field.

The diameter of the distal tip ranges from 14F to 16.2F; the tip may be blunted or tapered. The working length ranges from 37 to 40 cm and is approximately half the total length of the instrument. The range of distal tip deflection in one plane is 220° to 350°. Maximal deflection in one direction ranges from 180° to 220°, usually at the 12-o'clock position. Some tip deflection is lost when devices are passed along the working channel. The deflecting lever is on the handle near the eyepiece at the 6-o'clock position relative to the field marker. The irrigation working port enters on the opposite side of the endoscope. The flexible cystoscopes are immiscible for liquid sterilization, after which the working channel and entire cystoscope must be rinsed with sterile saline. If gas autoclaved, the instrument must be vented and aerated to protect its rubber components; this is done either by turning a knob on the handle or by connecting a vent attachment to the light cable before sterilization.

The irrigation working channel serves two purposes: the first is to provide for the flow of irrigant fluid and the second is to allow for the passage of instruments. Knowledge of the location

Table 1
Comparison of various flexible cystoscopes

Parameters	ACMI	Olympus	Storz	Wolf	Pentax
Model name/no.	ACN-2	8080072	11277A	730500	PCY-15P2
Features gas/soak valve	No—has auto seal	Yes	Yes	Yes	N/A
Head diameter (French)	15	16.2	15	15.5	14.4
Shaft diameter (French)	15.9	15.6	15	15.5	N/A
Working length (cm)	37	38	40	35	40
Depth of vision (mm)	3–50	2–50	3–50	2–50	3–50
Deflection angle	180° Up 170° Down	210° Up 90° Down	180° Up 14° Down	210° Up 90° Down	220° Up 90° Down
Working channel (French)	6.4	6.6	7.0	5.5	6.6
Field of view (H_2O)	110°	120°	120°	80°	83°
Detachable light cord	Yes	No	Yes	Yes	No

of the irrigation working channel port in the visual field is important for successful manipulation of instruments through the flexible cystoscope, as each brand of flexible cystoscope has a different location of port in regards to visual field. The diameter of the working channel is of critical importance. The larger the working channel, the better the better the flow of irrigant. The flow rate is approximately one fourth that of a similarly sized rigid cystoscope. If an instrument is placed through the working channel, it greatly decreases the flow rate, which is more profound with smaller working channels. To maintain flow when instruments are passed, it sometimes is necessary to increase the inflow pressure of the irrigant (raise the height of the irrigant reservoir or apply pressure cuff around the fluid bag) or use instruments of a smaller diameter.

Instruments placed through the working channel of the flexible cystoscope include stone baskets, grasping forceps, biopsy forceps, guide wires, electrocautery probes, electrohydraulic lithotripsy probes, laser fibers, flexible needles, and angiographic/ureteral catheters. The more flexible the instrument, the less the loss of tip deflection. In this regard, the biopsy forceps usually are the stiffest instruments, whereas the wire baskets and 3- or 4-prong graspers are the most malleable.

Technique for flexible cystoscopy

In the office, patients are asked to empty their bladder and are placed on examination table in the supine position. Then they are prepared and draped with the penis or urethra exposed. A topical anesthetic is instilled per urethra and left in situ for 5 to 10 minutes. The instruments necessary for office flexible cystoscopy are listed in Table 2.

Patients can be examined in almost any position; males can be examined in the supine position and females can be supine or frog legged. The flexible cystoscope is held in the dominant hand (Fig. 1), then the distal tip of the endoscope is inserted into the urethra. In male patients, the surgeon should grasp the penis with the fourth and fifth fingers of the nondominant hand and hold the penis erect and on a stretch (Fig. 2). The first three fingers are used to guide the endoscope along the urethra. In female patients, the endoscope is held by an assistant. The cystoscope is inserted into the urethra and advanced into the bladder. The entire urethra is viewed in a retrograde fashion. The field of view is that of a $0°$ lens.

Table 2
Instruments for office flexible cystoscope

- Flexible cystoscope
- Trays for sterilization by immersion and for rinsing the instrument after soaking in the sterilizing solutions
- Light source
- Irrigation tubing
- Normal saline for irrigations
- Penile clamp and 2% lidocaine for intraurethral anesthetic
- Sterile towels for draping the patient
- Betadine preparation solution
- 0.038-inch guide wire
- 5F olive tip catheter
- 5F biopsy forceps
- 5F alligator forceps
- 5F 3- or 4-prong grasping forceps

Optional
- Sorbitol or glycine for irrigation
- 0.038-inch torque guide wire
- 3F Bugbee electrocautery
- Electrocautery unit

If the field of view becomes obscured, it is likely that the endoscope is abutting the urethral mucosa. The endoscope should be pulled back until the urethral lumen is visible and the scope then should be advanced under direct visualization, especially at points of resistance (ie, at the external urethral sphincter and prostate). For diagnostic procedures, water or normal saline is adequate for irrigation. The scope should be deflected up to pass through the prostatic urethra. The bladder then should be inspected in a systematic fashion from dome to bladder neck (Fig. 3). Next the base of the bladder and trigone are inspected. Each ureteral orifice should be viewed and the character of the efflux (clear, bloody, or cloudy) should be noted. Finally, the endoscope is retroflexed upon itself to view the bladder neck (Fig. 4). This is done by deflecting the cystoscope fully and advancing the instrument into the bladder. The cystoscope curls on itself and provides an excellent view of the bladder neck. Median lobe hypertrophy and tumors at the bladder neck can be detected in this fashion [4]. The prostate should be examined in an antegrade fashion at the completion of cystoscopy. The bladder is inspected and finally the urethra is examined in an antegrade fashion.

One problem with flexible cystoscopes can occur in patients who have gross hematuria and clots or who have bladder debris. The decreased flow and small working channel of the instrument make visualization difficult and clot removal

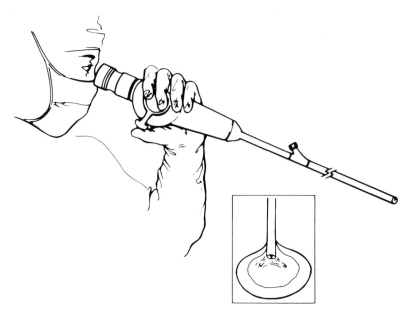

Fig. 1. The flexible cystoscope should be held in the dominant hand with the thumb resting on the deflecting leve, which should be facing the examiner's body. In this manner, when the examiner looks through the cystoscope, the field marker appears at the 12-o'clock position. (*From* Kavoussi LR, Clayman RV. Office flexible cystoscopy. Urol Clin North Am 1998;15:601–8; with permission.)

impossible. In this situation, the bladder should be irrigated clear by placing a large-bore catheter and irrigating out all clots or debris. In some cases, however, it may be more practical to perform rigid endoscopy [4].

Diagnostic and therapeutic procedures

Improvements in flexible instruments have changed the role of flexible cystoscopy from a purely diagnostic role to a powerful therapeutic tool [4]. A variety of therapeutic and diagnostic procedures can be done using the flexible cysto-scope. These include bladder biopsies, ablation of small bladder tumors, urodynamic evaluation for urinary incontinence, guide wire placement during difficult catheterizations, retrograde pyelography, placement of ureteral stents, removal of ureteral stents, and intraoperative consultations. This in-strument may be placed onto a cart containing a mobile light source; irrigating fluid and tubing; and numerous instruments, including wires, dila-tors, graspers, and catheters. This portable setup allows bedside treatment of a variety of urologic problems, including difficult catheterizations, stent manipulations, foreign body removal, and use for intraoperative consultations. The major

limitation is the inability to manage large bladder tumors properly.

A complete diagnostic flexible cystoscopic examination of the bladder can be performed in the office in fewer than 5 minutes using local anesthesia [2]. There is minimal discomfort to the patient with maximal information obtained. Also, patients who cannot be placed in a lithotomy

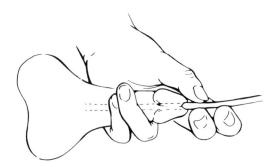

Fig. 2. Technique for performance of flexible cystoscopy in male patients. The penis is grasped in the fourth and fifth fingers of the nondominant hand, and the penis is held on the stretch. The first three fingers are used to guide the instrument into the urethra. (*From* Kavoussi LR, Clayman RV. Office flexible cystoscopy. Urol Clin North Am 1998;15:606; with permission.)

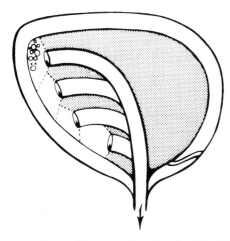

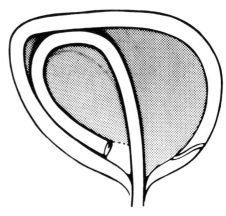

Fig. 3. Technique for systematic evaluation of the bladder. The entire bladder mucosa is examined with a field marker at 12-o'clock. The endoscope is deflected 90°s upwards until air bubble is seen. By withdrawing the endoscope to the bladder neck, all of the bladder along the 12-o'clock position is examined. (*From* Kavoussi LR, Clayman RV. Office flexible cystoscopy. Urol Clin North Am 1998;15:606; with permission.)

Fig. 4. The bladder neck is inspected by retroflexing the cystoscope. Small lesions at the bladder neck can be visualized and treated using this technique. With the field marker at 12-o'clock, the endoscope is deflected maximally in the upward direction, and advanced against the back wall of the bladder. The endoscope will curl upon itself, thereby revealing the bladder neck. (*From* Kavoussi LR, Clayman RV. Office flexible cystoscopy. Urol Clin North Am 1998;15:606; with permission.)

position, such as quadriplegics and paraplegics, patients in orthopedic casts, or patients who have severe arthritis, can be examined easily with the flexible cystoscope. The flexible cystoscope can be used to inspect the bladder through an existing suprapubic tract. Likewise, inspection of conduits can be performed more easily with a flexible cystoscope, as it can readily negotiate the full length of a tortuous ileal or colonic segment. In addition, male patients who have an elongated urethra secondary to penile prosthesis can be examined easily in the office. Several patients can be examined in one day, because the instrument can be liquid sterilized.

Surveillance cystoscopic monitoring in patients who have prior urothelial tumors is a primary indication for use of the flexible cystoscope. The entire surface of the bladder, including the bladder neck, can be inspected. Also, cytology samples can be obtained by barbotage with a 60-mL syringe connected to the working point of the flexible cystoscope. A 60-mL bolus of saline is instilled and withdrawn from the bladder four times as the body of the endoscope is rotated so the stream of irrigant can be directed toward the left lateral wall, right lateral wall, dome, and trigone. At the end of this procedure, as much saline as possible is aspirated for cytologic evaluation.

Suspicious lesions in the bladder can be examined by biopsy through the flexible cystoscope using 5F biopsy forceps. Samples are small, however, and may not be sufficient for diagnosis. Thus, to increase the diagnostic yield, multiple biopsies of a suspicious area should be obtained. The pathologist should be informed fully as to the size and location of the lesion.

When biopsies are obtained, a topical anesthetic agent (lidocaine 1% solution) is instilled into the bladder and left in place for 10 minutes before procedure. To perform a biopsy, the tip of the endoscope is placed within 3 mm of the lesion, and the biopsy forceps are extended until the back of the jaws is visible. The forceps then are opened and pushed into the lesion until it is visibly deformed. The forceps are closed tightly and either pulled through the endoscope or pulled out along with the endoscope. The latter maneuver yields a larger specimen. An electrocautery unit and a 3F or 5F electrocautery probe should be available for hemostasis. When cautery is used, the irrigant must be changed from saline to sorbitol or glycine.

As with the rigid endoscope, bladder outlet obstruction can be evaluated. Prostatic length can be estimated by pulling the endoscope just to the bladder neck, grasping the cystoscope with the first two digits of the nondominant hand at the meatus, and retracting the endoscope slowly until the verumontanum is reached. The distance from the examiner's fingers to the meatus represents the prostatic length. Other changes suggestive of bladder outlet obstruction, such as bladder trabeculation, cellule formation, and diverticular formation, also can be seen. Also, with the flexible cystoscope, urethral strictures and bladder neck contractures can be assessed. Likewise, vesical diverticula often can be inspected thoroughly for occult carcinoma.

Localization of the site of hematuria may be possible; however, in cases of macroscopic hematuria with clot formation, rigid cystoscopy in the operating suite under anesthesia is recommended. Lastly, evaluation of patients who have irritative voiding symptoms, interstitial cystitis, foreign body, or bladder calculus is possible with the flexible cystoscope.

When confronted with a difficult urethral catheterization, the flexible cystoscope allows direct visualization of the obstructing lesion (stricture, false passage, perforation, bladder neck contracture, or benign prostatic obstruction). Most of these lesions can be traversed with either the cystoscope or a standard 0.038-inch guide wire or glide wire placed through the working channel of the endoscope. If appropriate, the lesion then can be dilated in a stepwise fashion with sequential tapered urethral dilators. A Councill-tipped urethral catheter then may be placed over the guide wire. These same techniques also may be used when faced with inability to pass a catheter through a "catheterizable" stoma and for the replacement of a urethral catheter misplaced immediately after radical prostatectomy.

Ureteral stents can be placed and removed using flexible cystoscopy. Again, in this setting, the flexible cystoscope offers less discomfort and may be performed with the patient in the supine position obviating stirrups. A 5F alligator forceps be used to remove ureteral catheters. The stent is grasped and the cystoscope and stent are removed at the same time.

A flexible cystoscope with a 6F or larger working channel allows placement of ureteral stents under local anesthesia. This may be particularly useful immediately before shock wave lithotripsy in patients who are at risk for postoperative obstruction. In patients who have large renal pelvic or caliceal calculi, very hard calcium oxalate monohydrate calculi, narrow or tortuous ureteral anatomy, or solitary kidneys, the routine placement of ureteral stents should be considered.

A standard 0.038-inch guide wire is used to intubate the ureteral orifice and is advanced to the renal pelvis where resistance is encountered. A 4.8F double-pigtail ureteral stent then is advanced under direct visualization. Should the double pigtail fail to advance, a stiffer 6F open-end ureteral catheter may be tried in its place over the guide wire. The distal pigtail coil is verified endoscopically; proximal stent position may be verified with either a plain film radiograph or ultrasound. Fluoroscopy, if available, greatly facilitates this procedure.

Bladder biopsy under local anesthesia using the flexible cystoscope can be performed in an outpatient clinic setting and is an alternative to rigid cystoscopy and biopsy under general anesthesia. A specially designed, Teflon-insulated, 5.4F biopsy instrument is available, which can be passed through the 6F working channel of the flexible cystoscope and simultaneously can perform the bladder biopsy and tissue cauterization in one operation. Specimens thus obtained are shown to be satisfactory for tissue diagnosis, allowing transitional cell carcinoma, carcinoma in situ (cis), inflammatory processes, and normal bladder mucosa to be differentiated adequately. Minimal discomfort is associated with the biopsy portion of the examination. Lidocaine 2% jelly, instilled transurethrally or intravesically before biopsy, can decrease patient discomfort. If intravesical lidocaine jelly is used, the patient's bladder has to be emptied before cystoscopic examination. A careful cystoscopic examination is performed. Sterile water is used as the irrigation fluid. To obtain biopsies, an active electrical cord that adapts to the biopsy forceps and a standard electrocautery device are required. To obtain a biopsy, the forceps is advanced through the working port of the cystoscope. The area of interest is engaged with the jaws of the forceps under direct vision and just enough coagulating current is applied to the tissue to cause blanching of the surrounding urothelium. The cystoscope and specimen then are removed as a unit. The cystoscope can be reintroduced and further biopsies or fulguration can be performed. Small tumors at the bladder neck also can be treated using the flexible endoscope. Tumors at the bladder neck can be treated using either electrocautery using a 3F Bugbee electrode, Nd:YAG laser, or holmium:YAG laser. The ability of a flexible cystoscope to retroflex provides the surgeon the opportunity to reach tumors that may be difficult to address using rigid endoscopy.

With the availability of fluoroscopy tables in some urology offices, retrograde pyelography increasingly is performed using the flexible cystoscopy. It has an important role in selected cases for evaluating hydronephrosis, hematuria, and ureteric obstruction. The flexible cystoscope is passed into the bladder and a careful examination of the bladder is performed. After this, the scope is rotated through 180° to allow greater deviation of the tip of the scope and to facilitate identification of the ureteric orifices. Once the orifice of concern is identified, a 4F or 5F open-ended ureteral catheter is passed through the working channel into the bladder. A little amount of contrast then is injected through the ureteral catheter to clear any air bubbles that may be contained in it. The catheter then is used to intubate the ureteral orifice and contrast injected into upper urinary tract under fluoroscopy. Essential presurgery information can be obtained in this manner ahead of planned procedure.

A number of other procedures can be performed using the flexible cytoscope. These include urodynamic evaluation of the male external urethral sphincter, vaginoscopy, lithotripsy of bladder calculi, diathermy of small superficial bladder tumors, and evaluation of the bladder during surgical treatment of female incontinence. Most of these procedures require general anesthesia and are beyond the scope of office-based cystoscopy.

Genital condyloma

Human papilloma virus (HPV) infection is the most common sexually transmitted infection in young adults in the United States [5]. The clinical outcome of the infection is genital warts, predominantly caused by HPV types 6 and 11. Genital warts may cause additional symptoms of pain, bleeding, and itching, leading to perception of anxiety, fear of cancer, and, potentially, changes in sexual behavior [6–8].

Currently, the epidemiologic data, though not entirely clear, is estimated in approximately 500,000 to 1,000,000 new patient diagnoses in the United States annually. Furthermore, it is estimated that approximately 1% of sexually active adults have visible genital warts, whereas 15% have subclinical HPV [9]. Although treatment of genital warts places a substantial burden on the health care system, it is estimated that approximately 240,000 initial visits were the results of genital warts in 1999.

The larger verrucous papules are genital warts, also known as Condyloma acuminata. Conversely,

the small pearly papules on the corona are not warts but a variation of normal male anatomy called pearly penile papules. The rationale of recognizing these papules is to reassure men that they are normal and to avoid performing any invasive treatments to remove them.

A laboratory examination

All patients who have sexually transmitted disease should be treated for syphilis and HIV regardless of other risk factors [10].

Treatment

The primary treatment of visible genital warts is the removal of symptomatic warts. Treatment may induce wart-free periods and, at present, available therapies for genital warts may reduce, but probably not eradicate, infectivity. At present, no single treatment is ideal for all patients and all warts. The Centers for Disease Control and Prevention 2002 treatment guidelines for sexually transmitted diseases recommend the following options [10].

Patient-applied treatments

Treatment with podofilox 0.5% solution or gel is as follows: application of podofilox solution with a cotton swab or podofilox gel with a finger to visible genital warts twice a day for 3 days followed by 4 days of no therapy is recommended. This may be repeated up to a maximum of four cycles with appropriate counseling as to management and application of the solution or gel.

Imiquimod 5% cream

Patients should apply imiquimod cream once daily at bedtime 3 times a week for up to 16 weeks, with the treatment area washed with soap and water 6 to 10 hours after the application.

In-office management and treatment options include the following:

1. Cryotherapy with liquid nitrogen or cryoprobe, in repeated applications for 1 to 2 weeks, is recommended.
2. Podofilox resin 10% to 25% in a compound tincture of benzoin, with application to each wart followed by air dry, is recommended. The treatment should be repeated on a weekly basis. To avoid systemic absorption and toxicity, some specialists recommend that

application be limited to less than 0.5 mL per session.

3. A small amount of trichloroacetic acid is applied to the genital warts and allowed to dry, at which time a white frosting develops. This may be repeated weekly if necessary.

4. Surgical removal either by excision or a combination of excision and curettage or electrosurgery may be recommended.

In evaluating patients, it is helpful to note that the soft nonkeratinized warts respond well to the various forms of podofilox and trichloroacetic acid, although the keratinized lesions respond better to ablative methods, such as cryotherapy, excision, or electrocautery. Imiquimod works well for keratinized and nonkeratinized lesions.

A single randomized, multicenter, placebo-controlled study demonstrates that 0.5% podofilox gel is significantly better than placebo for successfully eliminating and reducing the number and size of anogenital warts [11]. In the intent-to-treat population, 37% treated with podofilox gel had complete clearing of the treated areas compared with 2% who had clearing of warts with the placebo gel after 4 weeks. Imiquimod has proved effective in many studies, including three randomized controlled trials, with clearance rates of 37% to 52% after 8 to16 weeks of treatment.

Recurrent rates for sole therapy with imiquimod (9% to 19%) are substantially lower than those for most other genital wart treatments, including podophyllotoxin.

Summary

Treatment options after appropriate evaluation and counseling are recommended for patients in an outpatient setting. For patients who have decided to use cryoablative approaches in the office, a prescription of imiquimod cream may be used for additional warts as well. Follow-up and sexual counseling are recommended for these patients and lead to ideal results on a long-term basis.

References

[1] Shah J. Endoscopy through the ages. BJU Int 2002; 89:645–52.

[2] Kavoussi LR, Clayman RV. Office flexible cystoscopy. Urol Clin North Am 1998;15:601–8.

[3] Goldfischer ER, Cromie WJ, Karrison TG, et al. Randomized, prospective, double-blind study of the effects on pain perception of lidocaine jelly versus plain lubricant during outpatient rigid cystoscopy. J Urol 1997;157:90–4.

[4] Beaghler MA, Stewart G, Dickinson MT. Update on flexible cystoscopy and nephroscopy. AUA Update Series 2002; XXI:Lesson 7.

[5] Kate W. Estimates of the incidence and prevalence of sexually transmitted diseases in the United States. American Social Health Association Panel. Sexually Transmitted Diseases 1999;26:S2–7.

[6] Griffiths TRL, Mellon JK. Human papillomavirus and urogenital tumors I: basic science and role in penile cancer. BJU Int 1999;84:579–86.

[7] Melbye M, Frisch M. The role of human papillomaviruses in anogenital cancers. Semin Cancer Biol 1998;8:307–13.

[8] Frisch M, Glimelius B, van den Brule AJ, et al. Sexually transmitted infection as a cause of anal cancer. N Engl J Med 1997;337:1386–8.

[9] Hippelainen MI, Syrjanen S, Hippelainen MJ, et al. Prevalence and risk factors of genital human papillomavirus infections in healthy males: a study on Finnish conscripts. Sex Transm Dis 1993;20:321–8.

[10] Centers for Disease Control and Prevention. Sexually transmitted diseases treatment guidelines. MMWR Recomm Rep 2002;51(RR-6):1–78.

[11] Tyring S, Edwards L, Cherry LK, et al. Safety and efficacy of 0.5% podofilox gel in the treatment of anogenital warts. Arch Dermatol 1998;134:33–8.

ELSEVIER
SAUNDERS

Urol Clin N Am 32 (2005) 327–335

UROLOGIC
CLINICS
of North America

Office-Based Prostate Procedures

Fatih Atug, MD, Erik P. Castle, MD,
Raju Thomas, MD, FACS, MHA*

*Department of Urology, Tulane University Health Sciences Center, 1430 Tulane Avenue,
SL-42, New Orleans, LA, USA*

Office-based procedures of the prostate consist primarily of treatments for benign prostatic hyperplasia (BPH). With the development of new technologies and the economic changes within the health care industry, invasive treatments for BPH have moved into the offices of urologists. Changes in reimbursement schedules coupled with consumer demand for minimally invasive treatment options have resulted in the development of a variety of office-based procedures for the treatment of symptoms secondary to BPH. The gold standard treatment always has been transurethral resection of the prostate (TURP). The voiding and quality-of-life benefits of TURP are well established within the urologic literature. The potential for significant intraoperative and postoperative complications, the need for hospital admission, and the associated costs, however, have stimulated the development of many minimally invasive alternatives. Treatments, such as transurethral microwave thermotherapy (TUMT), transurethral needle ablation (TUNA), intraprostatic injections, interstitial laser coagulation of the prostate, and urethral fluid balloon thermotherapy, are some of the available office-based treatments for BPH. This article reviews these developing therapeutic technologies for BPH. In addition, this article reviews the current prominent role of transrectal ultrasound (TRUS) of the prostate within the office setting.

Transurethral microwave thermotherapy

TUMT is a heat-based therapy offered to patients who have lower urinary tract symptoms (LUTS). It is considered an attractive treatment alternative to TURP because of its ease of administration and the minimal discomfort associated with it. TUMT treatment is based on increasing intraprostatic temperatures greater than 45°C, which cause coagulation necrosis in the targeted periurethral glandular tissue of the transition zone [1]. The heat is delivered through a catheter with a microwave antenna to selected portions of the prostate gland. Several devices are available, with the main differences between them being the degree of energy delivered, the cooling system, and design of the antenna.

Patient selection criteria

Inclusion
1. Refractory LUTS
2. Failed medical management of BPH
3. Urinary retention
4. Significant surgical and anesthetic risks

Exclusion
1. An obstructive median lobe
2. Urethral length less than 3 cm or greater than 5 cm
3. Prostate volume less than 30 g
4. Gross hematuria
5. Significant detrusor instability
6. Urethral strictures
7. Acute urinary tract infection
8. Acute prostatitis
9. Prostate or bladder cancer
10. Neurogenic bladder

---

* Corresponding author.
E-mail address: rthomas@tulane.edu (R. Thomas).

0094-0143/05/$ - see front matter © 2005 Elsevier Inc. All rights reserved.
doi:10.1016/j.ucl.2005.04.004

11. Previous pelvic or rectal surgery
12. Cardiac pacemaker or defibrillator implant
13. Pelvic or metallic implants

Recommended work-up

1. Cystoscopy
2. International prostate symptom score (I-PSS)
3. Urine flow studies
4. TRUS to assess urethral length
5. Postvoid residual assessment
6. Urodynamic evaluation if suspect a neurogenic component

Devices and manufacturers

1. Prostatron® (Technomed International, Lyon, France)
2. Targis® (Urologix, Inc., Minneapolis, MN)
3. Prostalund® (Lund, Sweden)
4. Prostcare (Spectrospin, Wissemburg, France)
5. TMx-2000 (Thermatrx, Northbrook, Illinois)
6. Urowave (Dornier Medical Systems, Wesling, Germany)
7. Prolieve Thermodilatation System (Boston Scientific Corporation, Natick, MA)

Procedure

All preoperative assessment is completed and patients are given detailed informed consent. Fleet enema is prescribed for the morning of treatment or three bisacodyl tabs are taken the afternoon before treatment. Local analgesia is administered with 10 mL of intraurethral 2% lidocaine jelly approximately 15 minutes before treatment. The bladder is emptied with a 16F red rubber catheter. After the bladder is emptied, 50 mL of 2% lylocaine solution is instilled for 10 minutes. Then, the TUMT catheter is placed into the bladder and the balloon is inflated. Positioning of the catheter balloon and antenna is confirmed by TRUS. The rectal probe for temperature assessment is inserted and treatment is commenced. Intramuscular analgesia, such as meperidine or anxiolytics, can be used for additional comfort before treatment. Treatment must be monitored at all times by a physician or another member of the urology team (Fig. 1).

Results

TUMT is effective in relieving LUTS and improving voiding parameters, according to

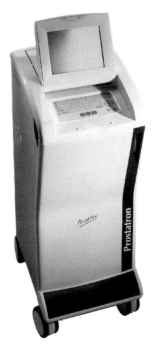

Fig. 1. Representative example of mobile TUMT equipment. (*Courtesy of* Urologix.)

studies with at least 1 year of follow-up [2–6]. In sham-controlled studies, symptom scores decreased between 40% and 70%, whereas peak urinary flow rates increased 14% to 60% [7–14]. The incidence of major complications associated with microwave treatment has been found substantially lower than that with TURP [15–18]. Prolonged postoperative catheterization times, urinary tract infections, and post-treatment irritative symptoms, such as dysuria, however, are the most common reported complications [19].

TUMT can be performed in an outpatient setting within an office without the need for anesthesiologists [14,20]. It can be performed in a single office session without general anesthesia or intravenous sedation. Djaven and coworkers demonstrate that TUMT is well tolerated by patients under topical anesthesia alone and can be administered in an outpatient setting without additional medications [20].

Transurethral needle ablation

TUNA of the prostate is another temperature-based minimally invasive treatment alternative for patients. Schulman and Zlotta first reported the feasibility of TUNA procedure in men who did not have LUTS resulting from BPH [21]. They conclude that this procedure can be performed safely in an outpatient setting and is effective for improving symptoms secondary to BPH.

TUNA uses the thermal properties of radio frequencies [22–28]. The TUNA catheter (Precision, VidaMed, Menlo Park, California) is fitted with two deployable needles angled 40° from each other. The needles deliver thermal energy by emitting 460- to 465-kHz signals from an automated generator that maintains a target temperature of more than 45°C at the periphery and approximately 100°C at the center. Coagulation necrosis can be achieved at a mean of 3 mm from the tip of the needles through agitation of water molecules causing friction and subsequent heat. Larger volume prostates may require multiple punctures to treat the area fully [29]. Depth of penetration by the deployed needles is preset and based on volume assessment and urethral length measurements. Furthermore, by controlling needle length with extendible Teflon (DuPont, Wilmington, Delaware) shields and varying generator wattage, unwanted injury to surrounding structures, such as the urethra and rectum, can be prevented (Fig. 2).

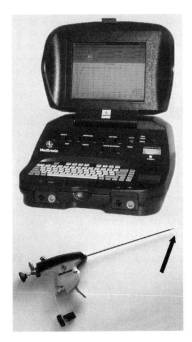

Fig. 2. The TUNA device—transurethral probe with needles extended (*arrow*), and the portable monitoring station. (*Courtesy of* Medtronic.)

Patient selection criteria

Inclusion
1. Refractory LUTS
2. Failed medical management of BPH
3. Urinary retention
4. Significant surgical and anesthetic risks

Exclusion
1. An obstructive median lobe
2. Gross hematuria
3. Significant detrusor instability
4. Urethral strictures
5. Acute urinary tract infection
6. Acute prostatitis
7. Prostate or bladder cancer
8. Neurogenic bladder

Recommended work-up
1. Cystoscopy
2. I-PSS
3. Urine flow studies
4. TRUS (to assess prostate dimensions for safe deployment of needles)
5. Postvoid residual assessment.
6. Urodynamic evaluation if a neurogenic component is suspected

Equipment

The TUNA device consists of a hand piece similar to a rigid 18F cystoscope with a 0° optical lens, a light source and irrigation system, a radio frequency generator that operates at a frequency of 460 to 465 kHz, and two deployable needles directed 40° from each other.

Procedure

Patients are taken to the procedure room and placed in the dorsal lithotomy position. After sterile preparation and draping, 2% lidocaine jelly is injected intraurethrally approximately 10 minutes before the procedure is initiated. When necessary, local anesthesia can be supplemented with oral or intravenous sedation. A broad-spectrum, prophylactic oral antibiotic is administered before the procedure. Under direct vision and with use of a 0° optical lens, the sheath is advanced and positioned in the prostate gland. The length of the needle deployment within the prostate is calculated from the transverse measurement of the prostate obtained during previous TRUS. The depth of the needle deployment is determined by subtracting 6 mm from the distance between the urethra and the prostatic capsule. Pathologic studies demonstrate that the thermal injury may extend 5 to 6 mm beyond the tip of the deployed needle; transversely, the lesions created during the ablation treatment may cover a distance of 10 mm. Simultaneously, the protective shields are deployed 5 to 6 mm over the shaft of the needle to protect the urethra. This last feature is one of the major advantages of the needle ablation technique, as it preserves the integrity of the urothelium and allows performance of the procedure with no or minimal discomfort to the patient.

When both needles are positioned appropriately in the prostate gland, the radio frequency energy is delivered with a power between 2 and 15 W for 5 minutes per lesion. The number of lesions created depends on the size of the prostate gland. One lesion (coagulation necrosis produced by the two needles) usually is performed per 20 g of prostate tissue. Depending on the size of the prostate gland (20 to 75 g), one to three planes of treatment (a lesion in the left and right sides of the prostate at the same level constitutes a plane) are created, beginning 1 cm from the bladder neck and continuing at 1.5-cm increments until approximately 1 cm proximal to the verumontanum. At the end of the procedure, the instrument is removed and the bladder is emptied. A catheter may or may not be placed routinely and patients are discharged home on the same day with 3 to 5 days of oral inflammatories and oral antibiotics.

Results

TUNA is a minimally invasive treatment option for patients who have LUTS secondary to BPH. In reports of up to 5 years of follow-up, TUNA is performed safely with symptomatic improvement in patients [30,31]. It reportedly is tolerated well by patients with only negligible discomfort and significant symptom score improvements [22–28,32]. There is a lower risk of adverse events compared with other more invasive treatments. Effects on sexual function are minimal, with lower rates of retrograde ejaculation and erectile dysfunction rates in approximately 3% of cases [30,33]. For patients desiring a minimally invasive treatment for BPH with minimal risk of bleeding and lower risk of sexual dysfunction, TUNA is an appealing alternative to TURP.

Prostatic tissue ablation

During the past 40 years, many investigators explored intraprostatic injection for the treatment of BPH. The goal was to reduce prostatic volume by necrosing, solubilizing, and eliminating prostate tissue. The main differences in the various techniques include the route of injection, the choice of the injectable agent, and patient indication. Injection routes include transurethral, transperineal, or transrectal approaches without the need for anesthesia [34,35]. The injection treatments were performed in an outpatient setting. Many different agents have been tried, with the majority reported to induce some degree of inflammatory response with eventual coagulative necrosis, subsequent shrinkage of the enlarged gland volume, and restoration of varying levels of voiding function.

Absolute ethanol represents the agent studied most widely and used clinically for in situ tissue ablation [35]. Another injectable agent previously investigated is hypertonic saline in liquid and gel form [33–37]. Hypertonic saline is found to ablate prostate tissue in murine and canine models. Few published studies, however, evaluate its clinical use. The use of botulinum toxin A, produced by the bacterium, Clostridium botulinum, recently has become popular for several indications in urology [38–40]. Most recently, its use has included intraprostatic injection for the treatment of BPH [38]. Although initially promising, reports are only in small numbers of patients with short-term follow-up.

Patient selection criteria

Inclusion

Similar to inclusion criteria for TUMT on the first page of this article.

Exclusion

1. Allergies to any of the injectable agents
2. Acute prostatitis
3. Acute urinary tract infection

Equipment

1. Inject Tx (InjecTx Inc., San Jose, California), a specially designed needle for injection of alcohol
2. Absolute ethanol in liquid form or viscous chemical gel (alcohol or hypertonic saline)

Results

Ethanol injection demonstrated encouraging results with regards to safety, symptom improvement, and prostate volume reduction [34,35,41]. The catheter usually was removed within 24 to 48 hours. American Urological Association symptom score and I-PSS improved rapidly, with 54% improvement after 6 months. All patients demonstrated improvements in flow rate (62%) and quality-of-life scores (35% to 40%) after 6 months. Urinary retention was not observed and no patient required subsequent surgery. There were no significant increases in patient serum concentrations of ethanol, sodium, and prostate specific antigen [35].

Absolute ethanol (AE) currently is under investigation for formal Food and Drug Administration approval as a new drug for the treatment of BPH (Investigational New Drug 61,337). This investigational study is a multicenter phase I/II trial, sponsored by American Medical Systems, currently ongoing within the United States [41].

Interstitial laser coagulation

Interstitial laser coagulation (ILC) of the prostate relies on the production and radiation of heat produced at a point source. Coagulation necrosis occurs deep inside the adenoma instead of at the prostatic urethra. Energy is delivered through a laser fiber introduced into the prostate.

Patient selection criteria

Inclusion and exclusion criteria are similar to the other minimal invasive treatment alternatives.

Equipment and manufacturers

1. Dornier MBB Medillas Fibertom 4060 (Dornier MBB Medizintechnik, Munich, Germany) is a neodymium:YAG– based system.
2. Indigo LASEROPTIC Treatment System (Indigo Medical Inc., Ethicon Endo-Surgery, Cincinnati, Ohio) is a diode laser fitted with a specially designed laser applicator [42,43].

Procedure

The laser fiber is through a cystoscope and inserted into the prostate through the prostatic urethra at an angle of 15° to 30°. Treatment consists of 1 or 2 punctures per 10 cm^3 of prostate tissue [29,42]. Under direct visual guidance, the laser fiber is inserted up to its depth marker. The amount of energy delivered is the primary treatment variable. Low-energy settings (5 to 7 W) create desired effects in approximately 10 minutes, whereas high-energy settings (20 to 50 W) may deliver treatment in seconds [42]. Areas of necrosis can be created up to 15 mm in diameter [29]. ILC

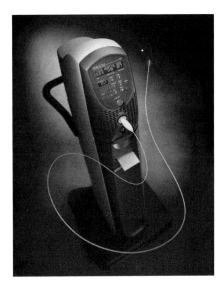

Fig. 3. ILC equipment with laser fiber attached. (*Courtesy of* Ethicon Endo-Surgery.)

can be performed with patients under local anesthesia in an outpatient setting (Fig. 3) [44,45].

Results

The catheter usually is removed within 2 to 7 days. Interstitial laser treatment of the prostate results in improvement of all clinical parameters but is inferior to improvement after TURP [46,47]. Operative complications are minimal, but the postoperative catheterization time is relatively long and irritative symptoms may last for a significant amount of time. The retreatment rates are high, 15% in 1 year, with reports as high as 40% in 3 years [47].

Advantages of ILC include the ability to treat asymmetric prostates, because the procedure can be adjusted by the surgeon cystoscopically [29]. ILC treatments can deliver deeper penetration and coagulation than other laser procedures. It can be performed repeatedly and spares the urethral mucosa, minimizing bleeding and discomfort [44].

Urethral fluid balloon–based thermotherapy

Another form of thermal-based tissue ablation is the use of hot water to heat the prostate conductively. The principle is to produce heat-induced coagulative necrosis and subsequent secondary ablation of obstructing hyperplastic tissue. Water-induced thermotherapy uses a closed looped catheter with two balloons. A proximal anchoring balloon within the bladder seats the catheter in place and a cigar-shaped treatment balloon stretches and treats the prostatic urethra [29].

Patient selection criteria

Inclusion criteria
1. Refractory LUTS
2. Failed medical management of BPH
3. Significant surgical and anesthetic risks

Exclusion criteria
1. Previous prostate surgery or other invasive prostatic treatments
2. Previous rectal surgery
3. A protruding median lobe

Manufacturers and equipment
1. Thermoflex (Argomed, Morrisville, North Carolina) water-induced thermotherapy system
2. Wallterm Fast Liquid Ablation System for Hyperplasia (FLASH) (Wallsten Medical SA, Morges, Switzerland) 5% dextrose solution

Procedure

Liquids, such as water or 5% dextrose solution heated at 60°C to 70°C, are circulated through the dilated treatment balloon. The remainder of the catheter shaft is insulated thermally to prevent damage to nontarget tissue. Temperatures ideally are limited to 43°C for the urethra and 42.5°C for the rectal wall. The Argomed system offers disposable catheters with treatment balloons ranging in sizes from 20 to 60 mm in 5-mm increments and can be performed in a single 45-minute office session with patients under only topical urethral anesthesia [48]. FLASH thermotherapy uses disposable treatment balloons that come in two sizes to fit eight lengths in 0.5-cm increments (2 to 3.5 and 4 to 4.5) and can be performed in an outpatient setting in 15 minutes.

Results

Urethral fluid balloon thermotherapy reportedly is tolerated well and indicated for treatment of BPH-associated LUTS. It does not, however, produce immediate tissue ablation and, therefore, requires postprocedural catheterization. Adverse effects of treatment include irritative voiding symptoms, such as urgency and dysuria [48–50]. In a prospective international study, the catheter was

removed after treatment when patients could achieve spontaneous voiding: 1 week in 45.5%, 2 weeks in 30.6%, and 3 to 5 weeks in 24.0% [48]. After 12 months, significant improvement was observed in I-PSS scores (48%), peak urinary flow rates (80%), and quality-of-life scores (37.5%). According to the literature, water-induced thermotherapy is a useful technique to treat BPH-related LUTS, with a success rate on an intent-to-treat basis of approximately 90% after 12 months and 75% after 24 months [49,50]. Physicians intending to use this technique are recommended to check on availability and regulatory matters before use.

Transrectal ultrasound of the prostate

TRUS of the prostate may be the most common office-based prostate procedure performed by urologists. It can serve as a diagnostic procedure for assessment of prostate volume and evaluation of prostate anatomy (ie, median lobe) and of surrounding structures, such as the seminal vesicles, or can be used to direct biopsies and treatment. The role of TRUS began having widespread application in the late 1980s, when it was combined with transrectal biopsy of the prostate to direct prostate sampling better [51].

TRUS is an excellent modality to assess prostate volume. Several reports compare digital rectal examination (DRE) to TRUS for prostate volume measurement and confirm its usefulness and improved accuracy in prostate volume estimation over DRE [52–54]. Some investigators find that DRE and TRUS size estimates are moderately to highly correlated in men who do not have prostate cancer [53]. Investigators point out, however, that DRE can underestimate size compared with TRUS, especially when prostate volume is more than 30 g [53,54]. More importantly, accurate measurement of prostate volume recently has received more attention because of findings from the Medical Therapy of Prostatic Symptoms study [55]. The benefits of combined medical therapy with α-blockers and 5α-reductase inhibitors seem greater in patients who have larger prostate volume and higher prostate specific antigens [56,57]. TRUS plays a role in the evaluation and work-up of BPH and LUTS.

TRUS is used by urologists primarily to direct prostate needle biopsies in the detection of prostate cancer. Prostate cancer is reported to be hypoechoic, hyperechoic, or isoechoic [58,59]. Because of this heterogeneity of possible appearances of cancer in the prostate gland, guided sampling techniques have evolved significantly. Some researchers have evaluated the usefulness of Doppler imaging, 3D and color, in prostate cancer detection [60]; however, the majority of prostate biopsies are performed with gray scale machines and specific sampling schemes. The exact number and most sensitive biopsy schemes are beyond the scope of this report, but the general consensus is to direct the biopsy needle into the lateral aspects of the prostate and take at least 4 to 6 cores from each side for a total of 8 to 12 cores [61]. Recently, periprostatic analgesia with lidocaine has gained popularity and injection of local anesthetic near the periprostatic nerves can be performed easily with ultrasound guidance [62–64]. TRUS has allowed for greater sensitivity in the detection of prostate cancer and improved patient comfort during prostate biopsy.

Soon after its usefulness in the setting of prostate biopsy was confirmed, the usefulness of TRUS in other areas was explored. TRUS can be used in the office setting to assist in the work-up of infertility. When ejaculatory duct obstruction is suspected, TRUS of the prostate potentially can identify dilated ejaculatory ducts or seminal vesicles [65,66]. Although TRUS can miss ejaculatory duct obstruction in the setting of low semen volume patients, it is a useful diagnostic tool before proceeding with transurethral surgery for infertility. TRUS can provide urologists with information on the anatomy and relationship of the seminal vesicle to the prostate. Prostatic cysts, calcifications, mullerian duct cysts, and the relationship to the rectal wall can be identified. Large median lobes even can be identified on TRUS. TRUS of the prostate is a useful diagnostic tool for practicing urologists when working up BPH, prostate cancer, or male infertility. In addition, TRUS is used in the preprocedure work-up of all the minimally invasive procedures (discussed previously).

Summary

The surgical treatment of symptoms secondary to BPH continues to evolve within the dynamics of current health care trends and economics. Medicare reimbursement schedules have changed over the past few years; hospital procedures have decreased whereas reimbursement has increased for office-based procedures [67]. Office-based procedures (described previously) and newer modalities will continue to find a place in the treatment of BPH. TURP is the gold standard with which all other modalities long will be compared. The

benefits of these minimally invasive treatments need to be weighed against the limitations of each treatment modality. Many of the available treatments have a decreased efficacy compared with TURP and some are associated with significant irritative voiding symptoms after treatment. The decreased risks associated with these treatments, however, such as bleeding, hyponatremia, and anesthetic risks, along with their use in outpatient settings, make them appealing to surgeons and patients. Furthermore, these alternate treatment options significantly expand urologists' armamentarium for the treatment of BPH. Being knowledgeable of the available treatment modalities and their advantages and inadequacies is vital in today's urologic practices. Finally, TRUS of the prostate will remain a crucial part of urologists' office-based practice.

References

[1] Roehrborn CG, Preminger G, Newhall P, et al. Microwave thermotherapy for benign prostatic hyperplasia with the Dornier Urowave: results of a randomized, double-blind, multicenter, sham-controlled trial. Urology 1998;51:19–28.
[2] Blute ML, Tomera KM, Hellerstein DK, et al. Transurethral microwave thermotherapy for management of benign prostatic hyperplasia: results of the United States Prostatron Cooperative Study. J Urol 1993;150:1591–6.
[3] Homma Y, Aso Y. Transurethral microwave thermotherapy for benign prostatic hyperplasia: a 2-year follow-up study. J Endourol 1993;7:261–5.
[4] Laduc R, Bloem FA, Debruyne FM. Transurethral microwave thermotherapy in symptomatic benign prostatic hyperplasia. Eur Urol 1993;23:275–81.
[5] Tubaro A, Paradiso Galatioto G, Trucchi A, et al. Transurethral microwave thermotherapy in the treatment of symptomatic benign prostatic hyperplasia. Eur Urol 1993;23:285–91.
[6] Marteinsson VT, Due J. Transurethral microwave thermotherapy for uncomplicated benign prostatic hyperplasia. A prospective study with emphasis on symptomatic improvement and complications. Scand J Urol Nephrol 1994;28:83–9.
[7] Bdesha AS, Bunce CJ, Kelleher JP, et al. Transurethral microwave treatment for benign prostatic hypertrophy: a randomised controlled clinical trial. BMJ 1993;306:1293–6.
[8] Ogden CW, Reddy P, Johnson H, et al. Sham versus transurethral microwave thermotherapy in patients with symptoms of benign prostatic bladder outflow obstruction. Lancet 1993;341:14–7.
[9] Bdesha AS, Bunce CJ, Snell ME, et al. A sham controlled trial of transurethral microwave therapy with subsequent treatment of the control group. J Urol 1994;152:453–8.

[10] de la Rosette JJ, de Wildt MJ, Alivizatos G, et al. Transurethral microwave thermotherapy (TUMT) in benign prostatic hyperplasia: placebo versus TUMT. Urology 1994;44:58–63.

[11] Mulvin D, Creagh T, Kelly D, et al. Transurethral microwave thermotherapy versus transurethral catheter therapy for benign prostatic hyperplasia. Eur Urol 1994;26:6–9.

[12] Blute ML, Patterson DE, Segura JW, et al. Transurethral microwave thermotherapy versus sham treatment: double-blind randomized study. J Endourol 1996;10:565–73.

[13] de Wildt MJ, Hubregtse M, Ogden C, et al. A 12-month study of the placebo effect in transurethral microwave thermotherapy. Br J Urol 1996;77:221–7.

[14] Larson TR, Blute ML, Bruskewitz RC, et al. A high efficiency microwave thermoablation system in the treatment of benign prostatic hyperplasia: results of a randomized, sham-controlled, prospective, double-blind, multicenter clinical trial. Urology 1998;51:731–42.

[15] Dahlstrand C, Geirsson G, Fall M, et al. Transurethral microwave thermotherapy versus transurethral resection for benign prostatic hyperplasia: preliminary results of a randomized study. Eur Urol 1993; 23:292–8.

[16] Kirby RS, Williams G, Witherow R, et al. The Prostatron transurethral microwave device in the treatment of bladder outflow obstruction due to benign prostatic hyperplasia. Br J Urol 1993;72:190–4.

[17] Dahlstrand C, Walden M, Geirsson G, et al. Transurethral microwave thermotherapy versus transurethral resection for symptomatic benign prostatic obstruction: a prospective randomized study with a 2-year follow-up. Br J Urol 1995;76:614–8.

[18] Eliasson TU, Abramsson LB, Pettersson GT, et al. Sexual function before and after transurethral microwave thermotherapy for benign prostatic hyperplasia. Scand J Urol Nephrol 1996;30:99–102.

[19] Walmsley K, Kaplan SA. Transurethral microwave thermotherapy for benign prostate hyperplasia: separating truth from marketing hype. J Urol 2004;172: 1249–55.

[20] Djavan B, Shariat S, Schafer B, et al. Tolerability of high energy transurethral microwave thermotherapy with topical urethral anesthesia: results of a prospective, randomized, single-blinded clinical trial. J Urol 1998;160:772–6.

[21] Schulman CC, Zlotta AR. Transurethral needle ablation of the prostate for treatment of benign prostatic hyperplasia: early clinical experience. Urology 1995;45:28–33.

[22] Chapple CR, Issa MM, Woo H. Transurethral needle ablation (TUNA). A critical review of radio-frequency thermal therapy in the management of benign prostatic hyperplasia. Eur Urol 1999;35: 119–28.

[23] Minardi D, Garofalo F, Yehia M, et al. Pressure-flow studies in men with benign prostatic hypertro-phy before and after treatment with transurethral needle ablation. Urol Int 2001;66:89–93.

[24] Namiki K, Shiozawa H, Tsuzuki M, et al. Efficacy of transurethral needle ablation of the prostate for the treatment of benign prostatic hyperplasia. Int J Urol 1999;6:341–5.

[25] Rasor JS, Zlotta AR, Edwards SD, et al. Transurethral needle ablation (TUNA): thermal gradient mapping and comparison of lesion size in a tissue model and in patients with benign prostatic hyperplasia. Eur Urol 1993;24:411–4.

[26] Roehrborn CG, Issa MM, Bruskewitz RC, et al. Transurethral needle ablation for benign prostatic hyperplasia: 12-month results of a prospective, multicenter US study. Urology 1998;51:415–21.

[27] Schatzl G, Madersbacher S, Djavan B, et al. Two-year results of transurethral resection of the prostate versus four 'less invasive' treatment options. Eur Urol 2000;37:695–701.

[28] Schulman CC, Zlotta AR. Transurethral needle ablation (TUNA): histopathological, radiological and clinical studies of a new office procedure for treatment of benign prostatic hyperplasia. Prog Clin Biol Res 1994;386:479–86.

[29] Blute ML, Larson T. Minimally invasive therapies for benign prostatic hyperplasia. Urology 2001; 58(6, Suppl 1):33–40.

[30] Hill B, Belville W, Bruskewitz R, et al. Transurethral needle ablation versus transurethral resection of the prostate for the treatment of symptomatic benign prostatic hyperplasia: 5-year results of a prospective, randomized, multicenter clinical trial. J Urol 2004; 171(6 Pt 1):2336–40.

[31] Zlotta AR, Giannakopoulos X, Maehlum O, et al. Long-term evaluation of transurethral needle ablation of the prostate (TUNA) for treatment of symptomatic benign prostatic hyperplasia: clinical outcome up to five years from three centers. Eur Urol 2003;44:89–93.

[32] Ramon J, Lynch TH, Eardley I, et al. Transurethral needle ablation of the prostate for the treatment of benign prostatic hyperplasia: a collaborative multicentre study. Br J Urol 1997;80:128–34.

[33] Larson BT, Bostwick DG, Corica AG, et al. Histological changes of minimally invasive procedures for the treatment of benign prostatic hyperplasia and prostate cancer: clinical implications. J Urol 2003;170:12–9.

[34] Larson TN, Palma P, Huidobro C. Controlled tissue ablation using chemo-gel injection under ultra-sound/MRI guidance. J Endourol 2001;Suppl A47: 11–2.

[35] Larson TN, Huidobro C, Palma P. Intraprostatic injection of ETOH gel for treatment of BPH: preliminary clinical results. J Endourol 2001;Suppl A132: 23–6.

[36] Adams J, Zvara P, Li S, et al., Hypertonic saline ablation for benign prostatic hyperplasia: an alternative to ethanol. Presented at the Annual Meeting of New

England Section of American Urological Association. Quebec City, Quebec, Canada, (p. 174 of abstract book) 2000.

[37] Lopes de LM, Ferreira U, Rodrigues NN Jr. Effect of hyperosmotic substances injected into the prostate of Wistar rats. J Endourol 2002;16:127–32.

[38] Maria G, Brisinda G, Civello IM, et al. Relief by botulinum toxin of voiding dysfunction due to benign prostatic hyperplasia: results of a randomized, placebo-controlled study. Urology 2003;62:259–64.

[39] Smith CP, Somogyi GT, Chancellor MB. Emerging role of botulinum toxin in the treatment of neurogenic and non-neurogenic voiding dysfunction. Curr Urol Rep 2002;3:382–7.

[40] Leippold T, Reitz A, Schurch B. Botulinum toxin as a new therapy option for voiding disorders: current state of the art. Eur Urol 2003;44:165–74.

[41] Plante MK, Folsom JB, Zvara P. Prostatic tissue ablation by injection: a literature review. J Urol 2004; 172:20–6.

[42] Muschter R, Whitfield H. Interstitial laser therapy of benign prostatic hyperplasia. Eur Urol 1999;35: 147–54.

[43] Mueller-Lisse UG, Thoma M, Faber S, et al. Coagulative interstitial laser-induced thermotherapy of benign prostatic hyperplasia: online imaging with a T2-weighted fast spin-echo MR sequence—experience in six patients. Radiology 1999;210:373–9.

[44] Volpe MA, Fromer D, Kaplan SA. Holmium and interstitial lasers for the treatment of benign prostatic hyperplasia: a laser revival. Curr Opin Urol 2001;11: 43–8.

[45] Zlotta AR, Schulman CC. Interstitial laser coagulation for the treatment of benign prostatic hyperplasia using local anaesthesia only. BJU Int 1999;83: 341–2.

[46] Martenson AC, De La Rosette JJ. Interstitial laser coagulation in the treatment of benign prostatic hyperplasia using a diode laser system: results of an evolving technology. Prostate Cancer Prostatic Dis 1999;2:148–54.

[47] Laguna MP, Alivizatos G, De La Rosette JJ. Interstitial laser coagulation treatment of benign prostatic hyperplasia: is it to be recommended? J Endourol 2003;17:595–600.

[48] Muschter R, Schorsch I, Danielli L, et al. Transurethral water-induced thermotherapy for the treatment of benign prostatic hyperplasia: a prospective multicenter clinical trial. J Urol 2000;164:1565–9.

[49] Muschter R. Conductive heat: hot water-induced thermotherapy for ablation of prostatic tissue. J Endourol 2003;17:609–16.

[50] Cioanta I, Muschter R. Water-induced thermotherapy for benign prostatic hyperplasia. Tech Urol 2000;6(4):294–9.

[51] Patel U. TRUS and prostate biopsy: current status. Prostate Cancer Prostatic Dis 2004;7:208–10.

[52] Loeb S, Han M, Roehl KA, et al. Accuracy of prostate weight estimation by digital rectal examination versus transrectal ultrasonography. J Urol 2005; 173:63–5.

[53] Roehrborn CG, Sech S, Montoya J, et al. Interexaminer reliability and validity of a three-dimensional model to assess prostate volume by digital rectal examination. Urology 2001;57:1087–92.

[54] Roehrborn CG, Girman CJ, Rhodes T, Hanson KA, Collins GN, Sech SM, et al. Correlation between prostate size estimated by digital rectal examination and measured by transrectal ultrasound. Urology 1997;49:548–57.

[55] McConnell JD, Roehrborn CG, Bautista OM, et al. The long-term effect of doxazosin, finasteride, and combination therapy on the clinical progression of benign prostatic hyperplasia. N Engl J Med 2003; 349:2387–98.

[56] Desgrandchamps F. Who will benefit from combination therapy? The role of 5 alpha reductase inhibitors and alpha blockade: a reflection from MTOPS. Curr Opin Urol 2004;14:17–20.

[57] Kim ED. The use of baseline clinical measures to predict those at risk for progression of benign prostatic hyperplasia. Curr Urol Rep 2004;5:267–73.

[58] Ellis WJ, Brawer MK. The significance of isoechoic prostatic carcinoma. J Urol 1994;152(6 Pt 2): 2304–7.

[59] Onur R, Littrup PJ, Pontes JE, et al. Contemporary impact of transrectal ultrasound lesions for prostate cancer detection. J Urol 2004;172:512–4.

[60] Inahara M, Suzuki H, Nakamachi H, et al. Clinical evaluation of transrectal power doppler imaging in the detection of prostate cancer. Int Urol Nephrol 2004;36:175–80.

[61] Romics I. The technique of ultrasound guided prostate biopsy. World J Urol 2004;22:353–6.

[62] Soloway MS. Do unto others—why I would want anesthesia for my prostate biopsy. Urology 2003; 62:973–5.

[63] Alavi AS, Soloway MS, Vaidya A, et al. Local anesthesia for ultrasound guided prostate biopsy: a prospective randomized trial comparing 2 methods. J Urol 2001;166:1343–5.

[64] Mallick S, Humbert M, Braud F, et al. Local anesthesia before transrectal ultrasound guided prostate biopsy: comparison of 2 methods in a prospective, randomized clinical trial. J Urol 2004;171(2 Pt 1): 730–3.

[65] Purohit RS, Wu DS, Shinohara K, et al. A prospective comparison of 3 diagnostic methods to evaluate ejaculatory duct obstruction. J Urol 2004;171: 232–5.

[66] Colpi GM, Negri L, Nappi RE, et al. Is transrectal ultrasonography a reliable diagnostic approach in ejaculatory duct sub-obstruction? Hum Reprod 1997;12:2186–91.

[67] Lotan Y, Cadeddu JA, Roehrborn CG, et al. The value of your time: evaluation of effects of changes in medicare reimbursement rates on the practice of urology. J Urol 2004;172(5 Pt 1):1958–62.

ELSEVIER
SAUNDERS

Urol Clin N Am 32 (2005) 337–352

UROLOGIC
CLINICS
of North America

Office Urologic Ultrasound

Sarah E. McAchran, MD[a], Vikram Dogra, MD[b],
Martin I. Resnick, MD[a],*

[a]Department of Urology, Case Western Reserve University School of Medicine, Cleveland, OH, USA
[b]Department of Imaging Sciences, University of Rochester Medical Center, Rochester, NY, USA

Until the introduction of cystoscopy and radiography in the late 1800s, sounding the bladder was one of the few methods of diagnosing a bladder stone. An office-based procedure, the bladder sound is introduced into a bladder filled with approximately 3 ounces of fluid [1]. Performing various manipulations of the sound, an entire bladder can be palpated, using the sound much the way a blind man uses his cane. When the sound discovers a stone, an audible click is heard. Although by no means flawless, sounding the bladder was one of the early ancestors of ultrasound (US) in urology. With US, a sound wave is emitted from the probe and travels into the body, where it encounters various surfaces and is reflected back to the US receiver, where that information is converted into a visual image.

The US machine is as integral to urologists' office at the dawn of the twenty-first century as the bladder sound was throughout the nineteenth century. Modern US machines are compact and portable and can be brought easily to the bedside, clinic, or operating room. Images are created in real time. Interpretation and diagnosis occur as the images are created. For these reasons, combined with the fact that US is completely noninvasive and without harmful side effects, US has been liberally adopted by urologists for its diagnostic and procedural capabilities. To obtain optimal images and make accurate clinical decisions, urologists must be trained in the use of basic US equipment and in US interpretation. This article reviews the basic physics behind US technology, optimal use of the equipment, and, finally, some of the more common uses of US in urology clinics.

Physics

Three basic principles of physics form the foundation for US technology. First, the piezoelectric effect describes the process by which piezoelectric crystals expand and contract to interconvert electrical and mechanical energy [2]. In 1880, Pierre and Jacques Curie observed that when pressure was applied to quartz crystals, an electrical charge was generated [3]. This charge was proportional to the force applied to it, and the phenomenon was called piezoelectricity.

In general, a transducer is any instrument that converts energy from one form to another. US transducers contain varying arrangements of piezoelectric elements, which consist most commonly of lead zirconate titanate ceramic embedded in a matrix of epoxy [4]. US pulses are formed by applying electrical waveforms to the piezoelectric element in the transducer, causing it to vibrate and emit US. Generating sound waves in the frequency range of 1 to 15 MHz, an US transducer directs these waves into the body where they are reflected, refracted, or absorbed. When reflected echoes return to the transducer resulting in vibrations, they are converted by the piezoelectric material into electrical signals, which then are amplified to produce an image. This illustrates the second basic physics principle, the pulse-echo principle, which states that when an US wave contacts a tissue, some of the signal is reflected back. The reflected waves detected by the transducer generate an

* Corresponding author. Department of Urology, Case Western Reserve University, 11100 Euclid Avenue, Cleveland, OH 44106-5046.
  E-mail address: martin.resnick@case.edu (M.I. Resnick).

0094-0143/05/$ - see front matter © 2005 Elsevier Inc. All rights reserved.
doi:10.1016/j.ucl.2005.03.005

electrical impulse comparable to the strength of the returning wave.

The third basic principle of US physics is acoustic impedance. Echo generation occurs when an US wave interacts with tissue. All tissues have a specific acoustic impedance that is determined by multiplying the density of the tissue by the speed of sound in the tissue. When US is directed at a homogenous fluid medium, such as a renal cyst, the sound waves are propagated without interruption and, thus, are not reflected back to the transducer, producing an anechoic (without echoes) image [5]. If the sound wave encounters a tissue of varying density, also called an acoustic interface, a portion is reflected back to the source and that area is visualized. The strength of the returning echo depends on, and is proportional to, the difference in density between the two structures imaged. For instance, the liver-kidney interface, representing two structures of similar density, emits weak echoes, whereas the interface between the fibrous renal capsule and the surrounding fat emits strong echoes, allowing it to be visualized discretely. Almost all sound is reflected at interfaces between air and soft tissue, necessitating the use of coupling mediums, such as gel, to prevent interference from intervening air pockets at the interface of the transducer and the skin.

When sound waves pass through soft tissue, only a small portion of the energy is reflected [4]. Most energy is attenuated by absorption, reflection, and scattering. Attenuation of US is the progressive weakening of the amplitude or intensity of the sound wave as it travels through a medium. It is measured in decibels and directly proportional to the frequency of the transducer used and the distance that the sound wave travels. Therefore, the higher the frequency (MHz), or the greater number of wave cycles per second, the greater the absorption by soft tissues, resulting in shallow penetration of the sound wave and higher attenuation. Wavelength is defined as the distance between two successive sound waves. Structures less than 1 wavelength apart cannot be detected as separate. Therefore, decreasing the US wavelength increases spatial resolution. Frequency and wavelength are related inversely, however, and as the wavelength is decreased to provide a more detailed image, the frequency is increased causing less soft tissue penetration. Conversely, as the wavelength is increased, the frequency decreases, providing deeper tissue penetration but sacrificing image resolution. Selecting a transducer with the appropriate frequency to best image the desired structure is critical to obtaining an optimal image. As a rule, it is best to select the highest frequency that permits adequate tissue penetration. For example, a 7.5- or 10-MHz transducer is used for scrotal US, whereas a 3- or 5-MHz transducer is used to view the kidneys (Table 1) [6].

Instrumentation

The basic US machine should include a hand-held probe or transducer, a pulse processing scanner, a monitor screen, and a recording device. Real-time scanning is a variant of B-mode US and is the mode with which most urologists are familiar. In real-time scanning, the tissue is scanned constantly and the display updated continually with many images per second, creating a real-time presentation. Special elements within the transducers are used to sweep sound waves repeatedly and rapidly through the tissue to be imaged, whereas the transducer head remains stationary [7]. This is called scanning. The pulse-processing scanner converts the US waves into a visual image that is displayed on the monitor. Each pixel on the screen represents the individual amplitude spike of a returning sound wave. With gray scale imaging, the brightness of the displayed dots is proportional to the intensity of the returning sound waves. Strong reflectors appear as bright white and are described as hyperechoic. Poor reflectors are darker shades of gray and are described as hypoechoic.

Most contemporary diagnostic US units are programmed with a variety of control presets, which make automatic adjustments for power, gain, time-gain compensation, contrast, focus, and depth [8]. Generally, US machine presets are changed automatically when a different transducer is used, for instance, when the transrectal probe is swapped for the bladder probe. Therefore, only minimal adjustments by the sonographer are required to obtain optimal images in most clinical scenarios. Power is the amount of US energy per unit of time transmitted from the US transducer. This should not require manipulation. The focus

Table 1
Transducer frequencies

Megahertz	
3.5–5.0	Kidney, bladder, transperineal
6.0–8.0	Prostate, seminal vesicles, urethra, transrectal, transvaginal
7.5–14	Scrotum, testicles, penis

and time-gain compensation are preset similarly. The gain control can amplify weak returning echoes so that a brighter image may be obtained. Increasing the gain effectively turns up the volume of an US image to improve clarity. Although depth generally is preset, some adjustments may need to be made to accommodate patients' body habitus or obesity.

The Doppler effect refers to the principle that if sound is reflected from a moving surface, the returning wave is at a different frequency from that of the transmitted wave. When applied to US, this shift in frequency can be detected and displayed visually in color or audibly and allows for the detection of blood and its direction of flow. Pulsed duplex Doppler US allows the operator to display the flow in an area on the corresponding gray scale image as a continuous time-velocity waveform [4]. Color Doppler US displays the color flow superimposed on a gray scale image, thus providing measurement of blood flow within specific blood vessels. Power Doppler US imaging is Doppler imaging without directionality. This makes the Doppler information stronger but with the loss of direction and quantitative velocity information [9]. It is 3 to 5 times more sensitive than color Doppler US and is of particular value in assessing small caliber vessels, such as the intrarenal arteries [10].

Innovations in image acquisition and processing further improves the depth and breadth of information attainable via B-mode and Doppler US [4,11,12]. Tissue harmonic imaging and spatial capture imaging provide crisper, more detailed displays by eliminating clutter and artifact [9,13]. Software packages make this technology readily available, even in the office setting. Coded pulse excitation allows deep structures to be imaged at higher frequencies, thereby improving spatial resolution at depth. With 3-D US reconstruction, algorithms create a 3-D image from a single sweep of the US beam [4,14]. These reconstructions allow unlimited viewing perspectives, more accurate volumetric measurements, and improved visualization of anatomic relationships. Finally, the use of contrast agents in US shows promise. These injectable agents are a fluid suspension containing small particles measuring 1 to 5 microns, which increase the back-scattered US signals, resulting in better image contrast [15]. They are used to characterize renal vascularity and renal masses [16]. US contrast agents are used in the office setting, in conjunction with color Doppler US, to target more accurately biopsies in prostate cancer [17,18].

Training

The American Urological Association (AUA) has developed guidelines for training and credentialing its members. The AUA policy statement, "Guidelines for Ultrasound Utilization," includes precise guidelines for instrument standards for prostate, renal, bladder, scrotal, and Doppler imaging, followed by a detailed list of the accepted indications for the use of US in urologic practice [19]. Educational requirements for US training during residency are delineated. For program accreditation, the Residency Review Committee for Urology requires training in the performance and interpretation of US; nine specific areas of mastery are described. The AUA believes that training in US should be hands-on and that "a cooperative effort between urologists and radiologists has proven to be an effective training methodology." The examination for certification by the American Board of Urology serves to assess the adequacy of resident training in US.

For those specialties that lack formal policies regarding training in diagnostic US, the American Institute of Ultrasound in Medicine (AIUM), the major professional society devoted to US, has developed training guidelines for physicians who evaluate and interpret diagnostic US examinations. The AIUM requires completion of a training program that includes at least 3 months of supervised diagnostic US training and evidence of the performance of 300 sonograms [20]. This number is increased to 500 for those physicians planning to use US for multiple subspecialty applications or anatomic areas. The American College of Radiology guidelines are the most stringent [21]. Nonradiologist physicians practicing US should have 200 hours of category I continuing medical education credits in the subspecialty in which they are performing US in addition to the documented performance of 500 supervised sonograms.

The AIUM also has published guidelines for standards of performance of the US examination of various organ systems, including the prostate, abdomen, and retroperitoneum, and scrotum. These standards include recommendations regarding necessary equipment, means of examination documentation and record keeping, and care of equipment. Furthermore, they describe the components included in the thorough examination of various structures. They assert that adherence to these standards is meant to maximize the detection of most abnormalities and serve as a standard of care. As an example, the standards set for prostate examination are: The prostate should be imaged in its entirety in at least two orthogonal planes, sagittal and axial or sagittal and coronal, from the apex to the base of the gland. In particular, the peripheral zone should be imaged thoroughly. The gland should be evaluated for size, echogenicity, symmetry, and continuity of margins. The periprostatic fat and vessels should be evaluated for asymmetry and disruption in echogenicity [22].

Nonradiologist physicians planning to bill for the performance and interpretation of diagnostic US should be well versed in these guidelines.

Kidney

Office examination of the kidney using US offers a quick evaluation of size, location, and shape. It can be performed to evaluate a variety of disorders: hydronephrosis, renal mass, renal calculus, and perirenal processes. A 3.5- to 5-MHz frequency, curvilinear or sector transducer is used to image the kidney. A thorough evaluation involves transverse and longitudinal US scanning with patients in supine and decubitus positions. With patients supine, the right kidney can be found by placing the transducer in the subcostal area at the anterior axillary line. The liver provides an acoustic window. The right lateral decubitus or posterior oblique position provides better access to the left kidney by avoiding overlying bowel gas, which dissipates the US beam. Posteriorly, the spleen provides the acoustic window.

The dense, fibrous renal capsule creates an acoustic interface with the surrounding fat. Thus, the renal outline is demarcated clearly on US (Fig. 1). In the transverse view, the kidney appears round. In the longitudinal view, the kidney appears elliptic with the upper and lower poles seen surrounding the renal sinus. The renal cortex appears as a region of homogenous low echogenicity. The renal sinus is echogenic and is seen as a dense echo complex consisting of peripelvic fat, renal and lymphatic vessels, and the normal collecting system. Optimally, the medullae are well differentiated from the cortex and appear as small, rounded, hypoechoic structures adjacent to the renal sinus. The medullae are more prominent in neonates than adults.

US is an excellent modality to determine renal size. Electronic rulers are superimposed on the renal images to determine the length of the kidney or any desired structure. The normal length of the

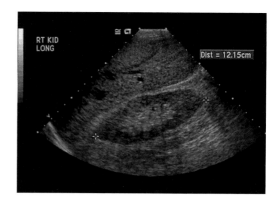

Fig. 1. Normal kidney, longitudinal view. The kidney appears elliptic with a homogenous renal cortex, which is hypoechoic compared with the echodense liver. The renal outline is well demarcated (within calipers) and the liver can be seen superiorly. (*From* McAchran SE, Dogra VS, Resnick MI. Office-based ultrasound for urologists. Part I: ultrasound physics, and of the kidney and bladder. AUA Update Series 2004;23 [lesson 28]; with permission.)

right kidney ranges from 8 to 14 cm and that of the left is 7 to 12.5 cm with sonographically obtained mean lengths of 10.74 and 11.0 cm, respectively.

Hydronephrosis

US is highly accurate in the diagnosis of hydronephrosis, with sensitivity ranging from 90% to 100% and specificity ranging from 90% to 98%. In the hydronephrotic kidney, the hyperechoic renal sinus is separated by the sonolucency of urine within the calices, infundibula, and renal pelvis, all in continuity (Fig. 2). As dilatation of the urinary tract progresses, the parenchyma and renal sinus are compressed. The amount of separation correlates with the severity of hydronephrosis. In extremely advanced hydronephrosis, the central echogenic sinus may be obscured completely [5].

Office-based US can be used to monitor the development, progression, or resolution of hydronephrosis in patients who have ureteral calculi and who are being observed for spontaneous passage. It also is invaluable in the postoperative period to monitor the development, progression, or resolution of urinary tract dilatation after extracorporeal shock-wave lithotripsy or other surgical procedures of the urinary tract, such as urinary diversion, ureteroneocystostomy, and

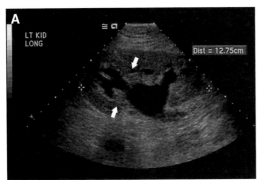 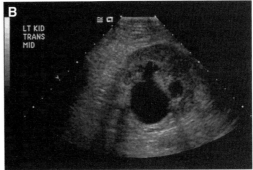

Fig. 2. Hydronephrosis, longitudinal (*A*) and transverse (*B*) views. Moderate dilatation of the calyces, infundibula, and renal pelvis is seen. Kidney size is enlarged slightly secondary to hydronephrosis (within calipers). (*From* McAchran SE, Dogra VS, Resnick MI. Office-based ultrasound for urologists. Part I: ultrasound physics, and of the kidney and bladder. AUA Update Series 2004;23 [lesson 28]; with permission.)

pyeloplasty. Furthermore, surveillance of patients who have urologic disorders that can progress to hydronephrosis is improved with regular US assessment [5]. Patients who have neurogenic bladders or bladder outlet obstruction and those who undergo urinary diversion can be assessed with US at regular office visits. If hydronephrosis develops or worsens, further evaluation and treatment can be undertaken.

Masses

US examination of the kidneys often is used as a noninvasive screening tool in the evaluation of patients who have microscopic hematuria. Simple renal cysts are the most commonly diagnosed pathology and US is capable of differentiating simple cysts from solid renal lesions, with an accuracy of greater than 98% [23]. US can detect cystic lesions that are only a few millimeters in diameter [5]. Solid masses are seen better when they approach at least 2 cm in diameter [24]. US criteria for the diagnosis of simple cysts are well established and include (1) anechoic structure, (2) well-defined back wall, (3) imperceptible cyst wall thickness, (4) enhanced posterior through-transmission, and (5) round or oval shape (Fig. 3). If these criteria are not met, the cyst is considered complex and further imaging is indicated. By providing better contrast and, in turn, better fluid-solid differentiation, tissue harmonic imaging likely aids in the more confident diagnosis of the simple cyst [13].

On US, solid renal masses usually are hypoechoic but can be hyperechoic in appearance. Solid masses attenuate US, do not demonstrate

enhanced through-transmission, have a poorly delineated posterior wall and demonstrate internal echoes (Fig. 4). Although US can differentiate between a solid mass and a cyst, it cannot differentiate benign masses from malignant masses. There are no characteristic features of renal cell carcinoma on gray scale, real-time B-mode US. When a solid or complex renal mass is found, the possibility of malignancy must be entertained and further evaluation is indicated. Contrast-enhanced multislice CT is the imaging modality of choice to characterize further these lesions. MRI may be used in patients who have

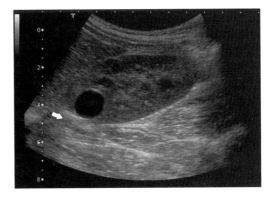

Fig. 3. Renal cyst, longitudinal view. The anechoic center is surrounded by crisp front and back and produces distal acoustic enhancement, or through-transmission (*arrow*). (*From* McAchran SE, Dogra VS, Resnick MI. Office-based ultrasound for urologists. Part I: ultrasound physics, and of the kidney and bladder. AUA Update Series 2004;23 [lesson 28]; with permission.)

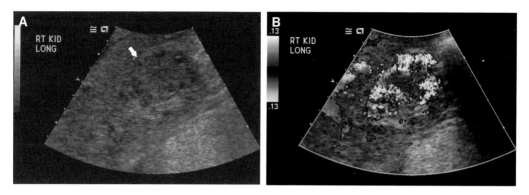

Fig. 4. Renal tumor, longitudinal view (*A*). This solid renal mass (*arrow*) has an echogenicity similar to that of the surrounding renal cortex. The margin with normal kidney is difficult to identify. When color Doppler is used, increased flow is seen in the area of the tumor (*B*). (*From* McAchran SE, Dogra VS, Resnick MI. Office-based ultrasound for urologists. Part I: ultrasound physics, and of the kidney and bladder. AUA Update Series 2004;23 [lesson 28]; with permission.)

poor renal function or radiographic contrast allergy. The presence of a cardiac pacemaker is an absolute contraindication for MRI.

Perirenal and renal pelvis processes

US is a sensitive modality for demonstrating perirenal fluid collections, such as lymphoceles, urinomas, hematomas, abscesses, and complications related to renal trauma. US cannot differentiate, however, among the different types of fluid collections. Finally, US can aid in the evaluation of noncalcified collecting system masses noted on intravenous pyelogram. A noncalcified renal calculus sonographically appears echodense and displays acoustic shadows (Fig. 5). Urothelial malignancies involving the upper urinary tract have a nonspecific, poorly echogenic sonographic appearance, and are difficult to distinguish from benign tumors, sloughed papilla, or blood clots.

Bladder

Bladder US can determine the presence and volume of postvoid residual urine; assess suspected bladder stones, diverticula, and other lesions; evaluate the bladder neck for hypermobility in women suspected of stress incontinence; and assess pediatric patients who have posterior urethral valves and ureteroceles.

Bladder US can be performed through a transabdominal, transrectal, transvaginal, or transurethral approach. Although evidence suggests that transurethral scanning may be the best method for

evaluation of bladder tumors, this approach requires the placement of a resectoscope sheath and does not lend itself to office use. When empty, the bladder lies behind the pubic symphysis and is difficult to find with US. Therefore, US should be performed with the bladder full. With patients supine, a 3.5-MHz transducer is placed 1 cm superior to the pubic symphysis and angled caudally. The bladder should be scanned in longitudinal and transverse orientations. In thin patients, a 5-MHz probe may provide adequate depth of

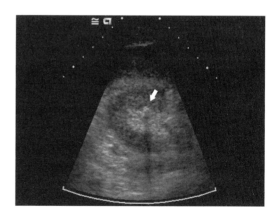

Fig. 5. Nephrolithiasis, transverse view. There is a bright echogenic focus (*arrow*) within the kidney, which demonstrates distal acoustic shadowing. This can be contrasted with the through-transmission seen in Fig 3. (*From* McAchran SE, Dogra VS, Resnick MI. Office-based ultrasound for urologists. Part I: ultrasound physics, and of the kidney and bladder. AUA Update Series 2004;23 [lesson 28]; with permission.)

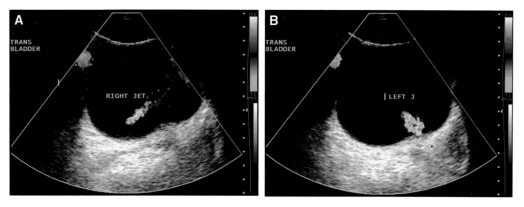

Fig. 6. Right (*A*) and left (*B*) ureteral jets. The flow of urine from the ureter into the bladder can be seen as a periodic echogenic foci emanating from the ureteral orifice. It is detected more easily if color Doppler is used, as shown here. (*From* McAchran SE, Dogra VS, Resnick MI. Office-based ultrasound for urologists. Part I: ultrasound physics, and of the kidney and bladder. AUA Update Series 2004;23 [lesson 28]; with permission.)

penetration and better resolution. In obese patients, a 2-MHz probe may be necessary [25]. Normal bladders have a smooth and symmetric thin wall and, when filled with fluid, are devoid of internal echoes. Sonographically, the individual layers of the bladder wall cannot be distinguished, and no consensus regarding normal maximal thickness has been reached. The shape of the bladder can vary with patient position and degree of distention. Sometimes the flow of urine into the bladder can be seen on routine US (Fig. 6). A ureteral jet of urine can be seen as an intermittent, echogenic focus emerging from the ureteral orifice. Ureteral jets are observed more easily with color flow Doppler [25].

Masses

Superficial transitional cell carcinoma appears as a polypoid, echogenic, or hyperechoic projection from the bladder wall [25]. Bladder disorders that can mimic malignancy on US include cystitis, bladder trabeculae, blood clots, stones, ureteroceles, and a prominent prostatic median lobe. The mobility of blood clots often distinguishes them from fixed neoplasms, but clots can be adherent. Bladder stones should move with changes in patient position and should appear hyperechoic with acoustic shadowing. The most common finding in cystitis is a diffusely thickened bladder wall. Ureteroceles have a fixed base with an anechoic center and thin echogenic wall (Fig. 7). The central location of a protuberant median prostate lobe usually helps to distinguish it from invasive bladder cancer.

Factors that affect the accuracy of transabdominal US in evaluating the bladder for malignancy include body habitus, bladder distention, and size and location of the tumor [25]. The dome and anterior bladder are difficult to evaluate with transabdominal US. The size of the tumors also is important, with studies noting diagnostic accuracy up to 38% for tumors smaller than 5 mm, 82% for tumors 5 to 10 mm, and 100% for tumors greater than 10 mm [26]. Transabdominal US also is less accurate in staging superficial versus deeply invasive tumors. In situ lesions cannot be detected and transabdominal US cannot distinguish Ta

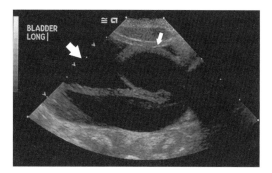

Fig. 7. Ureterocele, longitudinal view. The bladder is seen on the left (*large arrow*) and the ureterocele (*small arrow*) is seen on the right. It has the characteristic anechoic center and thin echogenic wall. The dilated ureter is seen inferiorly. (*From* McAchran SE, Dogra VS, Resnick MI. Office-based ultrasound for urologists. Part I: ultrasound physics, and of the kidney and bladder. AUA Update Series 2004;23 [lesson 28]; with permission.)

from T1 lesions or T1 from T2 lesions. If tumors have invaded beyond the bladder wall or involve the perivesical or retroperitoneal lymph nodes, transabdominal US can stage these lesions with an accuracy approaching 100% [27].

Residual urine

Measurement of residual urine is perhaps the most common application of bladder US in urologic office practice. US provides a rapid, noninvasive means to estimate residual urine volume without the risk of infection or the discomfort associated with urethral catheterization. Using the standard gray scale, real-time scanner, the bladder is imaged transversely and longitudinally. Measurements are taken of the width, height, and length. The equation for calculating the volume of an ellipsoid that is found the most accurate for estimating bladder volume is, volume $= 0.52 \times$ length $\times$ width $\times$ height. This calculation is performed automatically by most current US machines.

Newer devices or bladder scanners are small, portable, and designed specifically for automated bladder volume determinations by minimally trained personnel. The transducer is placed in the normal position for bladder US until the bladder shadow appears in the cross hairs of the sighting display. After activating the scanner, multiple US images spatially interlocked are generated at fixed angles to each other. A volumetric model of the whole bladder is constructed. Bladder volume is determined by a 3-D integration process rather than by a fixed geometric formula. Scanned volumes are shown to have an overall accuracy of 94% for volumes 100 mL or greater [28]. Scanned volume underestimates catheter volume by an average of 10 mL in men and 20 mL in women. The newest bladder scanners fit easily into the palm of a hand.

Urodynamics

Real-time US can be combined with standard urodynamics in the evaluation of voiding disorders and is proposed as a radiation-free alternative to fluoroscopy. Furthermore, US can provide useful information regarding the anatomy of the bladder base, pelvic floor, and urethra [29]. The bladder neck and proximal urethra are seen best via transrectal, transvaginal, and transperineal probe placement. For transrectal scanning, a high-frequency (7- to 10-MHz), linear array probe is preferred. Patients may be studied in the left lateral decubitus,

dorsal lithotomy, or standing positions. Once the probe is inserted, the face of the transducer is directed anteriorly toward the urethra. Transvaginal scanning is performed similarly. Transperineal scanning uses a 3.5- to 5.0-MHz probe placed on the perineum. On transverse section, three distinct layers of the urethra may be seen: an outer hyperechoic layer representing the rhabdosphincter, a central hyperechoic layer representing smooth muscle and connective tissue, and an innermost hypoechoic layer corresponding to the urethral lumen.

Transvaginal US is to evaluate the midurethra and urethral sphincter in cases of incontinence and urinary retention [30,31]. US measurement of the urethral angle is proposed for more accurate evaluation of urethral hypermobility [32,33]. Transperineal color Doppler US is used to measure urine velocity in the prostatic urethra of men who have bladder outlet obstruction [34,35]. Most of these applications still are in the experimental phase, and the widespread clinical applicability of US in this field remains to be determined.

Prostate

Transrectal imaging of the prostate may be performed to assess prostate size, locate focal abnormalities, calculate prostate specific antigen (PSA) density, and guide prostate biopsies. The office-based performance of US-guided prostate biopsies has become the primary modality used to diagnose prostate adenocarcinoma in patients who have an increased PSA or abnormal digital rectal examination. Biplane, multiplane, and endfire endorectal probes with a frequency range from 6 to 8 MHz are used to image the prostate and adjacent structures, including the seminal vesicles and urethra. When performing transrectal US examination, alone or in concert with prostate biopsy, the technique of examination is similar. A digital rectal examination is performed before the procedure to evaluate for anorectal abnormalities and palpate the prostate. With patients in dorsal lithotomy or lateral decubitus position, the well-lubricated transrectal probe is guided into the rectum above the anal verge. A systematic examination of the prostate and seminal vesicles is performed in transverse and longitudinal orientations, with pertinent images recorded and appropriately labeled.

The normal prostate appears homogeneous with a stipple gray echogenicity and a well-defined, echogenic, continuous capsule. The zonal anatomy usually can be identified. A distinct layer of echogenic fibrous tissue separates the transition zone from the central and peripheral zones. In transverse images, the prostate appears symmetric with a semilunar shape. The periurethral tissue can be identified as hypoechoic and centrally located, whereas the peripheral zone tissue has a fine, homogeneous echo pattern. In longitudinal or sagittal images, the relationship of the prostate to the bladder neck, seminal vesicles, and normal prostatic urethra easily is identified (Figs. 8 and 9). In the midline, the urethra appears as a curved structure within the central portion of the gland. Oriented horizontally in the transverse plane, the seminal vesicles are paired, symmetric, crescent-shaped structures that appear less echogenic than the prostate and are separated from the prostate base by hyperechoic fatty tissue.

Prostate volume

Measurement of prostate gland volume using US is accurate to within 5% of its true weight [36].

It is far more accurate than estimation by digital palpation. The length, width, and height of the prostate are measured using the transverse and longitudinal orientations. As with the bladder, the volume of the prostate then is estimated using the formula for an ellipsoid. Planimetry, which measures the surface area of the prostate at regular intervals throughout the gland and is used to determine gland volume, is the most accurate means of volume measurement. This method accommodates individual variations in prostate shape. With its superior accuracy, planimetry is used when planning brachytherapy treatment for prostate cancer.

Prostate volume is used in the calculation of PSA density, where serum PSA is interpreted in relation to prostate size. PSA density may help clinicians judge whether or not a PSA increase is the result of benign prostatic hyperplasia or malignancy. PSA density is calculated according to the equation, PSA density = PSA (ng/mL)/prostate volume (cm^3). A PSA density of 0.15 or greater is considered suspicious for cancer [6,37].

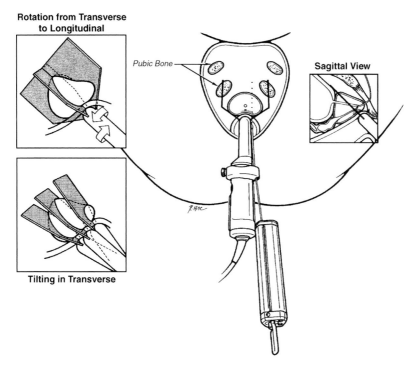

Fig. 8. Prostatic US and biopsy, transverse. The sound beam is directed from the tip of the biplanar, or end-fire, probe. Manipulating the probe in the anteroposterior direction images the prostate in transverse section from the apex to the base, as shown. (*From* Torp-Pedersen ST, Lee F. Transrectal biopsy of the prostate guided by transrectal ultrasound. Urol Clin North Am 1989;16:703; with permission.)

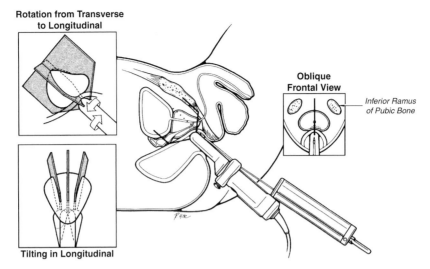

Rotation from Transverse to Longitudinal

Tilting in Longitudinal

Oblique Frontal View

Inferior Ramus of Pubic Bone

Fig. 9. Prostatic US and biopsy, longitudinal. Rotation of the probe 90° in either direction reaches the longitudinal plane. Angling the probe from left to right in this plane images the lateral borders of the prostate. (*From* Torp-Pedersen ST, Lee F. Transrectal biopsy of the prostate guided by transrectal ultrasound. Urol Clin North Am 1989;16:703; with permission.)

Prostate cancer

Exhaustive research has been aimed at determining the sonographic appearance of prostate cancer. It was hoped that transrectal US would be able to locate malignant lesions for biopsy and serve as a relatively noninvasive screening tool. Unfortunately, US proved disappointing in both regards [38]. The sonographic appearance of prostate cancer is varied, and early stage lesions tend to be indistinct from normal prostate tissue. Therefore, it has transpired that the true use of transrectal US resides in its ability to enable sampling of all relevant areas of the prostate, including those that appear normal ultrasonically [39].

The practice of systematic, sextant biopsies was described by Hodge et al in 1989 and remains the foundation of the prostate biopsy procedure [40]. The technical aspects of transrectal US-guided prostate biopsy are straightforward and ideally suited to urology offices. Before the procedure, patients should discontinue all anticoagulants. Recent studies demonstrate that prebiopsy cleansing enemas do not reduce the incidence of postprocedure infection significantly and can be abandoned [41]. Traditionally, 2 to 3 days of prophylactic antibiotics are prescribed but recent studies demonstrate that a single dose of a long-acting fluoroquinolone 1 hour before the procedure is sufficient antibiotic coverage and

does not increase the postprocedure infection rate of 1% [42–44].

With patients in a lateral decubitus or dorsal lithotomy position, a thorough sonographic examination of the prostate is performed. Suspicious, hypoechoic areas should be recorded. Periprostatic nerve blockade recently has been studied as a localized and uncomplicated method of decreasing the pain associated with prostate biopsy [25,45–48]. Under US guidance, a sterile 5-inch, 22-gauge spinal needle is passed through the biopsy needle port and positioned at the prostate base at the junction between the prostate and seminal vesicle—the site of the neurovascular bundle. Before injecting 2.5 mL of 1% lidocaine, the syringe is aspirated to ensure that intravascular injection does not occur, as this can cause seizures. Periprostatic nerve blockade is performed bilaterally.

A sterile 18-gauge biopsy needle is placed into a spring-loaded biopsy gun and advanced through the needle guide attached to the US probe. Using a marker line, available with most modern US view screens, any suspicious lesion can be biopsied in the sagittal or longitudinal plane. The rest of the prostate then should be sampled in a systematic fashion. There is considerable debate over the number and location of core biopsies necessary to detect prostate cancer, but the evidence suggests that an extended biopsy technique, including 10 to 12 cores and more laterally placed biopsies, improves detection over the traditional sextant technique [39,45,46].

Future

The roles of 3-D US and color and power Doppler US and the value of US contrast materials for the evaluation of prostate cancer are the subject of much current research [49]. In the future, all of these technologies may be available readily in urologists' offices. For tumors to grow, they require a blood supply. This blood supply is typified by low, slow flow. Power Doppler enables these small tumor vessels to be imaged by US in real time [25]. Color Doppler analysis is performed during transrectal US with a probe capable of color and pulsed Doppler. Advanced training in these techniques and their optimization is recommended. Increased flow in the peripheral gland is considered abnormal and suggestive of malignancy [47]. Interpretation of this increased flow, however, not always is straightforward, and the use of color Doppler US to increase sensitivity and specificity of transrectal US remains to be proven [48].

Two recent studies used intravenous US contrast in an attempt to enhance color Doppler US of the prostate [17,18]. As discussed previously, US contrast agents are injectable liquids that yield circulating microbubbles. These small air bubbles increase the echo density of the blood, resulting in enhanced visualization of the vasculature and better spatial resolution of the US image [48]. In both studies, contrast injection and color Doppler US were performed in the office setting, and there was encouraging improvement in biopsy sensitivity.

Similarly, 3-D US of the prostate can be performed easily in the office setting [50]. A 3-D endorectal volume transducer is substituted for the conventional 2-D US probe and can be coupled to a commercially available US unit. Automatic, planimetric volume scanning allows for nearly immediate reconstruction and display of sectional anatomy in orthogonal and oblique planes. As with all advanced US techniques, the examiner must be experienced with the operation of the system and with the interpretation of 3-D volumes. It remains to be proven, but 3-D US may be superior in depicting tumor presence and extraglandular extent of disease.

Scrotum

Scrotal US can be performed in the office to evaluate an enlarged or painful testis and to identify the gonad in the presence of a large hydrocele. Additionally, it can be used after trauma to evaluate a testicle for signs of rupture.

Complete scrotal examination involves the use of high frequency, small-parts transducers. Patients are supine and the probe is positioned on the scrotal skin using a coupling gel. While immobilizing the testicle with a free hand, images are taken in longitudinal, transverse, and oblique planes. The normal scrotal wall appears hypoechoic and is approximately 3 to 4 mm thick. A small amount of fluid between the visceral and parietal layers of the tunica vaginalis is common and appears as an anechoic area between the echogenic scrotal wall and testicle. The tunica albuginea usually is visualized only posteriorly, where it forms the mediastinum testis, and appears as an echogenic band of variable thickness and length parallel to the epididymis [51]. Sonographically, the testicle has a fine, uniform medium level echo pattern and measures approximately $5 \times 3 \times 2$ cm (Fig. 10). The epididymis, located posterolaterally to the testicle, is either hyperechoic or isoechoic compared with the testicle. Using color Doppler US, the testicular vessels can be identified in most patients [5]. Sonographic calculation of testicular volume, performed as described for the bladder and prostate, is more accurate than the traditional orchidometer and is recommended for any patient in whom testicular growth impairment is being evaluated [52].

Hydroceles

Hydroceles appear as anechoic regions surrounding the testicle. If fluid is present within the hemiscrotum, but this region contains echoes by

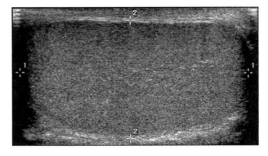

Fig. 10. Normal testicle, longitudinal. The normal testicle has a fine, medium level, homogeneous echo pattern. (*From* McAchran SE, Kogra VS, Resnick MI. Office-based ultrasound for urologists. Part II: prostate, scrotum, penis, urethra and office standards. AUA Update Series 2004;23 [lesson 29]; with permission.)

US, the fluid may represent a hematocele [51]. Spermatoceles are hypoechoic or anechoic and are differentiated from hydroceles by their location at the superolateral pole of the testicle. US is not needed to evaluate simple hydroceles or spermatoceles, as these entities have classic presentations on physical examination.

Masses

US is able to differentiate between intratesticular and extratesticular processes with great accuracy and has a near 100% sensitivity for detecting malignant testis tumors, most of which are hypoechoic, solid lesions. Seminomas tend to be homogeneous. Nonseminomatous lesions are more likely inhomogeneous because of internal hemorrhage, cystic changes, and calcification. Further differentiation is not the role of US, and surgical exploration is the procedure of choice if malignancy is suspected.

Acute scrotum

In an appropriate situation, US is a useful modality for evaluating patients presenting with acute scrotal pain and swelling. Despite continuing advancements in US technology, it still is recommended that patients who have a high likelihood of testicular torsion based on age, history, and physical examination undergo immediate surgical exploration. When the diagnosis of torsion is in doubt, however, color and power Doppler US provide a rapid, noninvasive method for evaluating the cause of an acute scrotum.

Acute epididymitis and epididymo-orchitis are the most common causes of acute scrotal pain. Gray scale US usually shows enlargement and hypoechogenicity of the involved epididymis and testis (Fig. 11). With new, high-frequency transducers, the presence of blood flow can be seen in the normal epididymis and, contrary to popular belief, the mere detection of blood flow in the epididymis is not diagnostic of epididymitis. Both epididymides should be compared side by side; relatively increased vascularity with increased concentration of vessels is suggestive of epididymitis [51]. The major complication of epididymitis is a testicular abscess, which can be seen as a focal testicular fluid collection with internal echogenic material.

In patients who have acute testicular torsion and an ischemic testicle, the testicle, as with acute epididymo-orchitis, appears enlarged and hypoechoic on US (Fig. 12). Therefore, color Doppler US must be used to distinguish torsion from inflammatory disorders. Color Doppler US demonstrates decreased or absent flow to the affected testicle compared with the normal contralateral testicle [53]. Power Doppler US is superior to color Doppler US for the pediatric testis because of the small-caliber vessels involved [54]. When performed properly, these studies are as reliable as radionuclide imaging and approach an accuracy of 98% [53].

Scrotal trauma

Testicular rupture is an uncommon sequela of blunt scrotal trauma. Sonographically, it appears

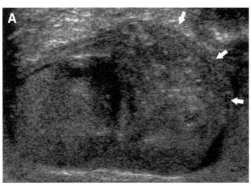 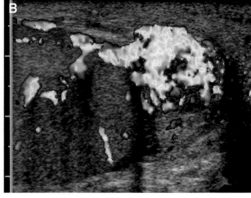

Fig. 11. Epididymitis, gray scale (*A*). The swollen epididymal head is shown (*arrows*). (*B*) Epididymitis; color Doppler imaging demonstrates the characteristic hyperemia of the epididymal head. (*From* McAchran SE, Kogra VS, Resnick MI. Office-based ultrasound for urologists. Part II: prostate, scrotum, penis, urethra and office standards. AUA Update Series 2004;23 [lesson 29]; with permission.)

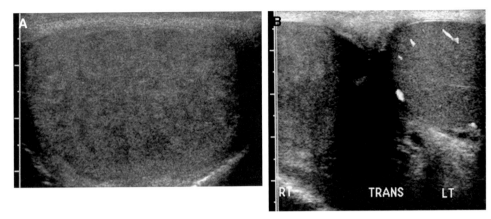

Fig. 12. Testicular torsion, gray scale (*A*). On gray scale image, the torsed testicle appears diffusely swollen and has a hypoechoic pattern. It does not appear significantly different from the testicle with epididymitis (Fig. 11A). (*B*) Testicular torsion, color Doppler. Only with color Doppler imaging can testicular torsion be diagnosed. Normal blood flow is seen in the left testicle, whereas an absence of Doppler flow is noted in the right, torsed testicle. (*From* McAchran SE, Kogra VS, Resnick MI. Office-based ultrasound for urologists. Part II: prostate, scrotum, penis, urethra and office standards. AUA Update Series 2004;23 [lesson 29]; with permission.)

as an interrupted tunica albuginea with extruded or fragmented testicular contents; however, a discrete fracture plane rarely is seen (Fig. 13) [55]. Typical findings include abnormal echogenicity in the testis, which corresponds to areas of hemorrhage and infarction. Because the accuracy of scrotal US in trauma remains variable, when US findings are indeterminate, patients should undergo immediate scrotal exploration [56].

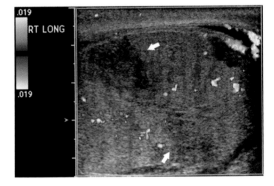

Fig. 13. Testicular fracture. Abnormal echogenicity within the testicle (*arrows*), which corresponds to the areas of hemorrhage and infarction. (*From* McAchran SE, Kogra VS, Resnick MI. Office-based ultrasound for urologists. Part II: prostate, scrotum, penis, urethra and office standards. AUA Update Series 2004;23 [lesson 29]; with permission.)

Penis and urethra

Penile US is performed with real-time scanning using high-frequency linear transducers (7 to 14 MHz). Color Doppler US is used to evaluate the penile vasculature. Patients are supine with the penis flaccid, resting against the anterior abdominal wall. Transverse and longitudinal images are obtained by positioning the probe on the ventral penis. The tunica albuginea and septum form a uniform hyperechoic border outlining the homogeneous cavernosum and spongiosum. The anterior urethra can be seen with the probe on the dorsal or ventral side of the penis. The bulbar urethra is imaged best with transperineal scanning. The posterior urethra is seen with transrectal US. Visualization of the urethra is facilitated by distention with saline or lidocaine jelly. The urethra is a hypoechoic luminal structure with an echogenic rim representing the mucosal/lumen interface.

Peyronie's disease

US is a rapid, noninvasive method for confirming the presence and extent of Peyronie's disease. Sonographically, Peyronie's plaque is represented by a thickened echogenic focus of tunica albuginea with areas of shadowing if calcification is present (Fig. 14). US can detect plaques before they are detectable on clinical examination. It also can be used to monitor the

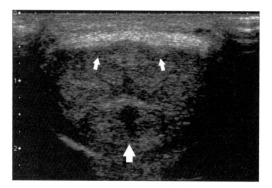

Fig. 14. Peyronie's plaque. In this transverse view of the penis, the small arrows are located in each corpora and are pointed to the thickened, echogenic focus of the tunica albuginea, which represents the plaque. The large arrow demonstrates the urethra with surrounding corpora spongiosum. (*From* McAchran SE, Kogra VS, Resnick MI. Office-based ultrasound for urologists. Part II: prostate, scrotum, penis, urethra and office standards. AUA Update Series 2004;23 [lesson 29]; with permission.)

response to treatment and the progression of the disease over time [57].

Urethra

Penile US provides accurate images of the anterior urethra [58]. The location and length of urethral strictures, associated degree of luminal narrowing, and associated fibrosis can be determined accurately. This information has prognostic importance and contributes to treatment planning. In the setting of acute trauma, the penis and urethra can be evaluated sonographically to identify areas of penile fracture and urethral disruption [59].

Urethral diverticula are an uncommon cause of lower urinary tract symptoms in women. Historically, voiding cystourethrography and double balloon urethrography were the diagnostic procedures of choice. MRI is shown to be sensitive but is cost prohibitive. Transvaginal US is suggested as a rapid, cost-effective, office-based assessment for urethral diverticulum [60]. The same high frequency probe that is used for transrectal US can be used for transvaginal US. The probe is inserted into the vagina until the bladder is identified. Moving caudally, and imaging in the transverse and sagittal planes, the urethra can be identified. A Foley catheter can be used to improve urethral visualization. The diverticula appears as a sonolucent fluid-filled mass near or adjacent to the urethra. Paraurethral cystic masses

that can be mistaken for urethral diverticula include Gartner's duct cysts, vaginal inclusion cysts, ectopic ureteroceles, endometrioma, and Skene's gland abscesses [25]. Demonstration of the communication between the cystic mass and the urethra confirms the diagnosis.

Summary

US should be performed by appropriately trained clinicians. Various definitions of appropriate training are proposed. Office-based, urologist-operated US is not intended to replace evaluation of patients by radiologists who are trained specifically to make diagnoses using this modality. For quick, efficient evaluation of patients to uncover disease process or to monitor the progress thereof, however, office US may supplement the information available through routine history, physical examination, and laboratory studies.

References

[1] Joly JS. Stone and calculous disease of the urinary organs. St. Louis: C.V. Mosby; 1929.
[2] Rozycki GS. Surgeon-performed ultrasound: its use in clinical practice. Ann Surg 1998;228:16–28.
[3] Newman PG, Rozycki GS. The history of ultrasound. Surg Clin North Am 1998;78:179–95.
[4] Hangiandreou NJ. AAPM/RSNA physics tutorial for residents. Topics in US: B-mode US: basic concepts and new technology. Radiographics 2003;23:1019–33.
[5] Spirnak J, Resnick MI. Ultrasound. In: Gillenwater JY, Grayhack JT, Howards SS, Mitchell ME, editors. Adult & pediatric urology. 4th edition. Philadelphia: Lippincott, Williams & Wilkins; 2002. p. 123–50.
[6] Horstman W, Watson L. Ultrasound of the genitourinary tract. In: Resnick MI, Older RA, editors. Diagnosis of genitourinary disease. 2nd edition. New York: Thieme; 1997. Chapter 6.
[7] Kremkau F. Doppler ultrasound: prinicples and instruments. Philadelphia: WB Saunders; 1990.
[8] Smith RS, Fry WR. Ultrasound instrumentation. Surg Clin North Am 2004;84:953–71 [v.].
[9] Strang J. Ultrasound physics. In: Dogra V, Rubens D, editors. Ultrasound secrets. Philadelphia: Hanley & Belfus; 2004. p. 1–7.
[10] Hamper UM, DeJong MR, Caskey CI, et al. Power Doppler imaging: clinical experience and correlation with color Doppler US and other imaging modalities. Radiographics 1997;17:499–513.
[11] Harvey CJ, Pilcher JM, Eckersley RJ, et al. Advances in ultrasound. Clin Radiol 2002;57:157–77.
[12] Whittingham TA. New and future developments in ultrasonic imaging. Br J Radiol 1997;70:S119–32.

[13] Schmidt T, Hohl C, Haage P, et al. Diagnostic accuracy of phase-inversion tissue harmonic imaging versus fundamental B-mode sonography in the evaluation of focal lesions of the kidney. AJR Am J Roentgenol 2003;180:1639–47.

[14] Downey DB, Fenster A, Williams JC. Clinical utility of three-dimensional US. Radiographics 2000;20:559–71.

[15] Deng C. Contrast agents for ultrasound imaging. In: Dogra V, Rubens D, editors. Ultrasound secrets. Philadelphia: Hanley & Belfus; 2004. p. 23–9.

[16] Robbin ML, Lockhart ME, Barr RG. Renal imaging with ultrasound contrast: current status. Radiol Clin North Am 2003;41:963–78.

[17] Roy C, Buy X, Lang H, et al. Contrast enhanced color Doppler endorectal sonography of prostate: efficiency for detecting peripheral zone tumors and role for biopsy procedure. J Urol 2003;170:69–72.

[18] Frauscher F, Klauser A, Volgger H, et al. Comparison of contrast enhanced color Doppler targeted biopsy with conventional systematic biopsy: impact on prostate cancer detection. J Urol 2002;167:1648–52.

[19] American Urological Association. Policy statement: guidelines for ultrasound utilization. Available at: www.auanet.org. Accessed: March 2005.

[20] American Institute of Ultrasound in Medicine. Training guidelines for physicians who evaluate and interpret diagnostic ultrasound examinations. Available at: www.aium.org. Accessed: March 2005.

[21] Grant E, Barr LL, Borgstede J, et al. American College of Radiology. Practice guideline for performing and interpreting diagnostic ultrasound examinations. Available at: www.acr.org. Accessed: March 2005.

[22] Hobbins J. Standards for performance of the ultrasound examination of the prostate (and surrounding structures). Available at: www.aium.org. Accessed: March 2005.

[23] Pollack HM, Banner MP, Arger PH, et al. The accuracy of gray-scale renal ultrasonography in differentiating cystic neoplasms from benign cysts. Radiology 1982;143:741–5.

[24] Jamis-Dow CA, Choyke PL, Jennings SB, et al. Small (< or = 3-cm) renal masses: detection with CT versus US and pathologic correlation. Radiology 1996;198:785–8.

[25] Cochlin DL, Dubbins PA, Goldberg BB, et al. Urogenital ultrasound: a text atlas. Philadelphia: JB Lippincott; 1994.

[26] Malone PR. Transabdominal ultrasound surveillance for bladder cancer. Urol Clin North Am 1989;16:823–7.

[27] Singer D, Itzchak Y, Fischelovitch Y. Ultrasonographic assessment of bladder tumors. II. Clinical staging. J Urol 1981;126:34–6.

[28] Marks LS, Dorey FJ, Macairan ML, et al. Three-dimensional ultrasound device for rapid determination of bladder volume. Urology 1997;50:341–8.

[29] Kuo HC. Transrectal sonographic investigation of urethral and paraurethral structures in women with stress urinary incontinence. J Ultrasound Med 1998;17:311–20.

[30] Kondo Y, Homma Y, Takahashi S, et al. Transvaginal ultrasound of urethral sphincter at the mid urethra in continent and incontinent women. J Urol 2001;165:149–52.

[31] Wiseman OJ, Swinn MJ, Brady CM, et al. Maximum urethral closure pressure and sphincter volume in women with urinary retention. J Urol 2002;167:1348–51 [discussion 1351–2].

[32] Pregazzi R, Sartore A, Bortoli P, et al. Perineal ultrasound evaluation of urethral angle and bladder neck mobility in women with stress urinary incontinence. Br J Obstet Gynaecol 2002;109:821–7.

[33] Reddy AP, DeLancey JO, Zwica LM, et al. On-screen vector-based ultrasound assessment of vesical neck movement. Am J Obstet Gynecol 2001;185:65–70.

[34] Ozawa H, Kumon H, Yokoyama T, et al. Development of noninvasive velocity flow video urodynamics using Doppler sonography. Part I: experimental urethra. J Urol 1998;160:1787–91.

[35] Ozawa H, Kumon H, Yokoyama T, et al. Development of noninvasive velocity flow video urodynamics using Doppler sonography. Part II: clinical application in bladder outlet obstruction. J Urol 1998;160:1792–6.

[36] Hastak SM, Gammelgaard J, Holm HH. Transrectal ultrasonic volume determination of the prostate–a preoperative and postoperative study. J Urol 1982;127:1115–8.

[37] Benson MC, Whang IS, Olsson CA, et al. The use of prostate specific antigen density to enhance the predictive value of intermediate levels of serum prostate specific antigen. J Urol 1992;147(3 Pt 2):817–21.

[38] Shinohara K, Wheeler TM, Scardino PT. The appearance of prostate cancer on transrectal ultrasonography: correlation of imaging and pathological examinations. J Urol 1989;142:76–82.

[39] Klein EA, Zippe CD. Transrectal ultrasound guided prostate biopsy—defining a new standard. J Urol 2000;163:179–80.

[40] Hodge KK, McNeal JE, Terris MK, et al. Random systematic versus directed ultrasound guided transrectal core biopsies of the prostate. J Urol 1989;142:71–4 [discussion: 74–5].

[41] Carey JM, Korman HJ. Transrectal ultrasound guided biopsy of the prostate. Do enemas decrease clinically significant complications? J Urol 2001;166:82–5.

[42] Terris MK, McNeal JE, Stamey TA. Ultrasonography and biopsy of the prostate. In: Walsh PC, Retik AB, Vaughan ED, et al, editors. Campbell's

urology. 8th edition. Philadelphia: WB Saunders; 2002. p. 3038–54.

[43] Aron M, Rajeev TP, Gupta NP. Antibiotic prophylaxis for transrectal needle biopsy of the prostate: a randomized controlled study. BJU Int 2000;85: 682–5.

[44] Griffith BC, Morey AF, Ali-Khan MM, et al. Single dose levofloxacin prophylaxis for prostate biopsy in patients at low risk. J Urol 2002;168:1021–3.

[45] Scherr DS, Eastham J, Ohori M, et al. Prostate biopsy techniques and indications: when, where, and how? Semin Urol Oncol 2002;20:18–31.

[46] Eskew LA, Bare RL, McCullough DL. Systematic 5 region prostate biopsy is superior to sextant method for diagnosing carcinoma of the prostate. J Urol 1997;157:199–202 [discussion: 202–3].

[47] Rifkin MD, Sudakoff GS, Alexander AA. Prostate: techniques, results, and potential applications of color Doppler US scanning. Radiology 1993;186: 509–13.

[48] Aarnink RG, Beerlage HP, De La Rosette JJ, et al. Transrectal ultrasound of the prostate: innovations and future applications. J Urol 1998;159:1568–79.

[49] Goldman SM, Sandler CM. Genitourinary imaging: the past 40 years. Radiology 2000;215: 313–24.

[50] Hamper UM, Trapanotto V, DeJong MR, et al. Three-dimensional US of the prostate: early experience. Radiology 1999;212:719–23.

[51] Dogra VS, Gottlieb RH, Oka M, et al. Sonography of the scrotum. Radiology 2003;227:18–36.

[52] Diamond DA, Paltiel HJ, DiCanzio J, et al. Comparative assessment of pediatric testicular volume: orchidometer versus ultrasound. J Urol 2000; 164(3 Pt 2):1111–4.

[53] Burks DD, Markey BJ, Burkhard TK, et al. Suspected testicular torsion and ischemia: evaluation with color Doppler sonography. Radiology 1990; 175:815–21.

[54] Barth RA, Shortliffe LD. Normal pediatric testis: comparison of power Doppler and color Doppler US in the detection of blood flow. Radiology 1997; 204:389–93.

[55] Corrales JG, Corbel L, Cipolla B, et al. Accuracy of ultrasound diagnosis after blunt testicular trauma. J Urol 1993;150:1834–6.

[56] Fournier GR Jr, Laing FC, McAninch JW. Scrotal ultrasonography and the management of testicular trauma. Urol Clin North Am 1989;16: 377–85.

[57] Hamm B, Friedrich M, Kelami A. Ultrasound imaging in Peyronie disease. Urology 1986;28: 540–5.

[58] Nash PA, McAninch JW, Bruce JE, et al. Sono-urethrography in the evaluation of anterior urethral strictures. J Urol 1995;154:72–6.

[59] Kervancioglu S, Ozkur A, Bayram MM. Color Doppler sonographic findings in penile fracture. J Clin Ultrasound 2004;33:38–42.

[60] Gerrard ER Jr, Lloyd LK, Kubricht WS, et al. Transvaginal ultrasound for the diagnosis of urethral diverticulum. J Urol 2003;169:1395–7.

ELSEVIER SAUNDERS

Urol Clin N Am 32 (2005) 353–370

Office Urodynamics

Emily E. Cole, MD, Roger R. Dmochowski, MD, FACS*

Department of Urologic Surgery, A-1302 Medical Center North, Vanderbilt University Medical Center, Nashville, TN 37232, USA

The field of urodynamics (UDS) has evolved significantly since its conceptual inception in the early twentieth century. The first urodynamic instrument, the cystometrograph, designed for measurement of bladder pressure during filling and voiding, was introduced in 1927 by Rose [1]. This instrument soon was followed by the uroflowmeter, measuring urinary flow rate, which was introduced to clinical practice in 1948 by Drake [2]. In 1956, von Garrelts expanded on the introductory uroflowmeter, developing an electronic version, which calculated the rate of flow based on increasing weights of urine collected over time [3]. In 1955, Franksson and Peterson introduced the first entry into the field of neurourology, the use of electromyography (EMG) to measure the muscular activity in response to voiding [4]. Visualization of the lower urinary tract during voiding first was introduced via cinefluoroscopy by Hinman and Miller in 1954 [5]. This concept of cinefluoroscopy was integrated with pressure-flow studies and then with urethral pressure profilometry by Miller [6] and was expanded on further by Turner-Warwick and Whiteside in London in the 1970s [7].

This period of conceptual development was followed by a phase of commercialization, during which urodynamic equipment was refined and mass produced, becoming available in office settings to most urologists. The indications, practices, and available equipment are evolving continually; however, the knowledge and basic concepts behind UDS studies remain much the same as when they first were developed.

UDS is a general term for a collection of techniques performed in an attempt to qualify and quantify the lower urinary tract activity during two fairly discrete phases of micturition: filling and storage, and emptying. Conceptually, normal, efficient bladder filling and storage require five components: (1) bladder compliance (distensibility); (2) bladder stability; (3) competence of ureterovesical junctions (ie, nonrefluxing ureters); (4) competent, closed vesical outlet at rest and during times of increased intra-abdominal pressure; and (5) appropriate bladder sensations. Bladder emptying requires (1) a coordinated contraction of bladder smooth muscle of adequate magnitude; (2) a synergic lowering of resistance at the level of the smooth and striated sphincter; and (3) the absence of obstruction. Any abnormality of filling and storage or of emptying, regardless of causative pathophysiology, must result from a problem related to one of these factors. UDS studies can assist in categorizing and quantifying these problems [8].

UDS studies are a combination of noninvasive measures, such as initial uroflowmetry, and invasive measures, such as filling cystometrogram. With the evolution of the personal computer has come much development in the field of UDS. The advent of smaller, less cumbersome, and less expensive machines has expanded the availability of complex UDS, including videourodynamics (VUDS), to more practicing urologists. This discussion broadly reviews the fundamental concepts behind technique, application, and interpretation of UDS testing and how they are applicable to general urologists in office settings. Some of this discussion is based on the authors' experience and

---

* Corresponding author.

E-mail address: roger.dmochowski@vanderbilt.edu (R.R. Dmochowski).

0094-0143/05/$ - see front matter © 2005 Elsevier Inc. All rights reserved.
doi:10.1016/j.ucl.2005.04.007

that of others in the field. A basis for these opinions and more in-depth discussions may be found in several reference texts [9–11].

Indications

Generally, UDS studies provide an objective tool with which physiologic information about the function of the lower urinary tract can be obtained and used in the diagnosis and management of bothersome conditions. It generally is accepted that patient-reported lower urinary tract symptoms correlate poorly with objective findings on UDS in all patient populations [12–15]. This, however, does not obviate the importance of UDS testing but rather underscores the lack of specificity of patient-reported lower urinary tract symptoms [16]. Although it is the symptoms that initially bring patients into physicians offices, the desire to uncover the pathophysiology responsible for these symptoms to guide treatment more appropriately is one of the main forces driving the use of UDS testing.

Because UDS are not designed as a substitute for a thorough history, physical examination, voiding diary, pad test, and other noninvasive testing, there remains unending debate regarding the appropriate application of this testing modality. In general, most urologists agree that UDS is indicated in those patients when a diagnosis cannot be made reliably using less invasive means of evaluation and in those cases when potential harm could result from a missed or mistaken diagnosis [17]. In addition, it is the authors' practice to perform UDS testing in all patients in whom irreversible, expensive, or potentially morbid procedures are considered for treatment of certain conditions and in patients in whom invasive interventions have failed to correct the presenting problem or have resulted in de novo complaints. In these circumstances, UDS testing can characterize and quantify certain complaints further and confirm a diagnosis before the use of invasive therapeutic measures.

When considering the use of UDS testing in patients without the absolute indications discussed previously, the benefit versus cost, inconvenience, and morbidity of tests must be considered. The complication rate of UDS, although generally minor, reportedly is as high as 19% [18]. Reported complications include urinary tract infection, urosepsis, urethral trauma from catheterization, and urinary retention [19]. As a result of these factors and economic considerations, many physicians and patients may choose empiric therapy for voiding dysfunction and defer definitive UDS testing as a part of initial evaluations. Some argue that if empiric therapy is successful, the cost and potential morbidity of the test can be avoided and that in cases of failure, UDS testing can be used [20]. Others argue that initial UDS testing assists in arriving at an accurate initial diagnosis and guiding appropriate therapy, avoiding the costs of potentially multiple empiric therapeutic interventions and the resultant prolonged patient suffering. In some patients, the decision to pursue initial invasive evaluation with UDS testing involves physician and patient comfort levels regarding the certainty of initial noninvasive diagnosis and the potential adverse outcomes or anxiety about empiric therapy [8].

Other potential indications of UDS evaluations include a role in risk stratification and prognosis for certain disorders; predicting the response to planned treatment, thereby facilitating preintervention counseling; demonstrating reasons for failed treatments; confirming the effects of specific treatments; and guiding therapy in complex voiding dysfunction patients.

Initial approaches

Initial evaluation of patients who have lower urinary tract symptoms includes an accurate history, physical examination, and a variety of noninvasive objective measures, such as pad test, voiding diary, postvoid residual, and so forth. After initial assessment, a working diagnosis is formulated and the need for further, more invasive testing is determined. In cases in which UDS is planned as a part of the evaluation, the working diagnosis should be able to be refuted or denied on completion of the study. UDS is not a substitute for other components of the initial evaluation.

UDS or VUDS studies are in most cases performed by clinicians or by skilled nurses or technicians under the supervision of clinicians. Ideally, UDS tracings should be interpreted by clinicians performing the studies. Particularly in cases when this is not practical, UDS studies should be labeled appropriately with patient information, history, physical examination findings, and all results of prior testing. Events and timing during the studies must be recorded accurately on the UDS tracing to allow for accurate future interpretation.

The primary goal during UDS studies is to reproduce patient symptoms during performance of a study. If examiners are unable to reproduce presenting symptoms or problems, then studies may be worthless. In these cases, it is recommended that examiners redo the study, reevaluate the diagnosis, or reconfigure the testing environment to perform more accurate studies. UDS studies are performed under artificial circumstances. The unfamiliar, technical, and invasive testing environment may serve to inhibit or disinhibit normal lower urinary tract function. Patients are asked to report sensations and to urinate outside the comfort and without the privacy provided by their own homes. Furthermore, patients go through these studies with urethral and sometimes rectal catheters in place, attached to a variety of tubes and monitors, adding to their potential discomfort. Cystometrogram is performed by filling the bladder at supraphysiologic rates with nonphysiologic solutions, both of which have potential for inducing or suppressing involuntary detrusor contractions. Catheterization of the urethra may be traumatic or painful, a factor that can suppress the micturition reflex [21].

These issues emphasize the importance of appropriate patient selection, excellent technique, meticulous interpretation, and an understanding of the potential pitfalls that can confound test results.

Equipment

There is considerable variability in the currently available setups for UDS with or without video capability. Several companies offer urodynamic equipment of different complexities, varying in cost, size, portability, adaptability, and compatibility with imaging modalities (fixed fluoroscopic units, portable C-arm fluoroscopic units, ultrasound units, and so forth). An example of a set-up using a fixed fluoroscopic unit is shown in Fig. 1, and an example using C-arm capability is shown in Fig. 2.

Uroflowmetry

The simplest portion of UDS studies arguably is the initial uroflowmetry phase. A standard uroflow, based on a measurement of urine volume passed per time unit, has been used in clinical practice for many decades. The measured urinary flow is a product of detrusor contractility combined with outlet resistance and can be modified

with abdominal straining, providing only a measure of total voiding function. It is the authors' practice to perform uroflowmetry on all patients before beginning multichannel UDS. Patients are asked to report to the office with a full bladder and then directed to void freely into a container during which a number of variables are graphically and electronically recorded (Table 1). The flow curve is characterized by the shape, the maximum flow (Qmax), the time to Qmax, and the flow time (Fig. 3). From the data obtained, the average flow rate can be calculated and a volume-corrected Qmax can be estimated from Qmax/square root of the voided volume. Finally, the ratio of Qmax to time to Qmax can be calculated to describe the flow acceleration from void initiation to Qmax. Generally, flowmeters are sufficiently precise for clinical practice when volume (error 1% to 8%) and flow (error 4% to 15%) are considered [22–24].

The peak and mean urine flow rates along with the flow pattern usually are considered the most commonly used and most reliable electronically recorded variables. If these parameters are normal, it is unlikely that there is a significant disorder of emptying. As the uroflow does not couple detrusor pressures with flow, however, a normal flow rate and pattern do not exclude the presence of pathology, particularly obstruction. Abnormal flow patterns come only in a few varieties. Consistently low, unbroken flow curves with asymmetry and an elongated, flattened course from Qmax to the end of voiding generally indicate increased outlet resistance, impaired contractility, or both. A specific diagnosis cannot be confirmed without information about the detrusor pressures during this flow pattern. Flow rates considerably in excess of normal may indicate decreased outlet resistance. A fractionated, discontinuous flow curve generally is secondary to abdominal straining or increased activity of pelvic floor muscles or sphincteric complex during voiding but may be representative of multiple low amplitude detrusor contractions.

The primary factor of importance when interpreting uroflowmetry and attempting to relate results with symptoms and diagnosis is that a test must correlate as much as possible with a typical voiding event for a patient. As discussed previously, uroflowmetry should be performed before the inception of the more invasive phase of the UDS test and should be performed under the most natural circumstances possible. It is reported that there is a significant dependence of flow rate on

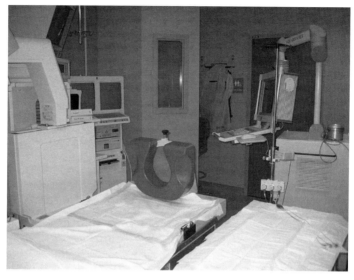

Fig. 1. Office VUDS set-up using fixed fluoroscopic unit.

volume voided, and it is recommended that voided events of less than 100 to 150 mL should be interpreted with caution [22,25]. Correlation with a voiding diary may be helpful in estimating a patient's functional bladder capacity and in determining the usefulness of the uroflowmetry test.

Although flow rates in large cohorts of patients generally are reproducible, there is considerable intraindividual variability when events are recorded sequentially [26,27], an important consideration when evaluating patients on multiple occasions.

In men, a Qmax of greater than 15 mL per second is considered normal, whereas a Qmax of less than 10 mL per second is considered abnormal [28]. These normal values, however, were determined by studies involving men under the age of 55 [29,30]. These studies and others demonstrate that Qmax declines with increasing age in symptomatically normal patients [30–34]. The significance of this is unknown, as these

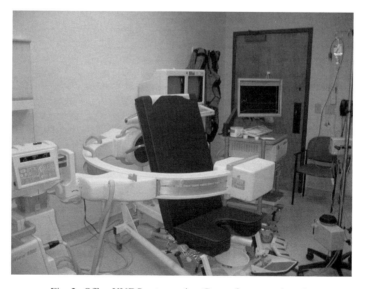

Fig. 2. Office VUDS set-up using C-arm fluoroscopic unit.

Table 1
Uroflow study: recorded values

- Flow pattern
- Voided volume
- Qmax
- Flow time
- Average flow rate
- Time to Qmax

values are not correlated with concomitant detrusor pressures to determine the impact of bladder outlet obstruction.

Assigning normal values in females is more difficult. In women, uroflowmetry is characterized by the shorter urethra and no resistance, such as that caused by the prostate gland in the male. Thus, the only factor influencing the normal female uroflow is the voluntary part of the sphincteric mechanism. Normal values are described as a Qmax between 20 to 36 mL per second [35–40]. The flow curve typically is bell shaped and the flow time is shorter than in men. There is no report of variability dependent on age. Further investigation is necessary to establish standardized minimum acceptable values for each gender and for various age groups.

Although there are considerable limitations to uroflowmetry, it is cheap, fast, and noninvasive and may provide practicing urologists with information that may direct toward or against

further, more invasive testing. In addition, it may serve as a useful, cost-effective method of following patients after medical or surgical interventions.

Postvoid residual volume

It is the authors' practice to measure a catheterized, postvoid residual urine volume after uroflowmetry. The advent of small, portable, ultrasonographic machines allows postvoid residual volume to be determined in a noninvasive and reproducible manner. Noninvasive residual volume determination is common practice in most settings and increasingly is used. Additionally, reimbursement now exists for this modality.

The amount of urine remaining in the bladder after a normal voiding event can provide useful information about the interplay of the bladder and the outlet during emptying. The definition of a normal postvoid residual volume is subject to controversy. In adults, it is suggested that a value of less than 25 mL is considered normal and one greater than 100 mL warrants careful surveillance or treatment. Some suggest that in certain circumstances, for example in the elderly, a postvoid residual volume of greater than 100 mL is acceptable [41].

As with uroflometry, considerable intraindividual variability may occur with sequential evaluations over time. Simple generalizations, however, can be made about lower urinary tract

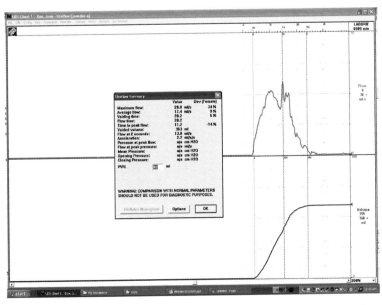

Fig. 3. Example of a normal uroflow. (Courtesy of Laborie Medical Technologies, Burlington, VT.)

function based on residual volume. Rovner and Wein state, "a consistently and significantly elevated residual urine volume is indicative of relative detrusor failure (impaired contractility), with or without concomitant bladder outlet obstruction. Conversely, negligible residual urine is compatible with normal function of the lower urinary tract; however, it may also exist with significant disorders of filling or storage or emptying disorders in which the intravesical pressure is sufficient to overcome increases in outlet resistance up to a certain point" [8].

Filling cystometry

Cystometry remains the most accurate tool for evaluating the passive filling component of bladder function. This phase of UDS studies is invasive and requires urethral or suprapubic catheterization. The goal of cystometry is the reproduction of patients' clinical status to improve diagnosis and guide therapy. As with other components of the UDS evaluation , the information obtained from cystometry should be integrated with that obtained from the patient's history, physical examination, voiding diary, and other preliminary studies.

The technique of cystometry can affect the overall results and must be followed in a standardized fashion to optimize interpretation of studies and to allow cross-comparison between studies. Multichannel pressure recording allows simultaneous measurement of multiple variables. Two types of materials are used for cystometric studies: gas and liquid. Carbon dioxide cystometry allows rapid performance of a study, with a relatively cost-effective material. Carbon dioxide, however, remains a relatively nonphysiologic infusant and is shown to induce bladder instability with even standard filling rates. Additional disadvantages to the use of carbon dioxide include the inability to measure leak-point pressures and the inability to assess the voiding phase of the micturition process. Liquid cystometry uses sterile water, normal saline, or contrast material as the infusant. Liquid cystometry is believed more physiologic because the infusant approximates the physical properties of urine. Other advantages include the ability to determine pressure-related fluid loss, estimate leak-point pressures, substantiate the presence of incontinence, and allow for subsequent evaluation of the voiding phase of micturition. In addition, when contrast medium is used as the

infusant, radiographic equipment may be used to assess the lower urinary tract anatomically during various stages of the UDS evaluation. Characteristics of the liquid can affect cystometric parameters, namely inducing or suppressing involuntary detrusor contractions [42,43].

The International Continence Society has established criteria for the standardization of filling rates during cystometry [44]. Under most circumstances, filling is performed at medium fill rate (10 to 100 mL per minute). Slower rates can be used in patients who have demonstrated significant instability or hyperreflexia at a faster fill rate. Provocative filling is performed using rates greater than 100 mL per minute. Rates of this magnitude can induce occult instability and are useful for evaluating patients who have significant urgency [45].

Cystometry can be performed with varying degrees of sophistication, depending on the equipment available. Bedside cystometry can be performed by attaching a 50-mL syringe to a urethral catheter and holding it 15 cm above the symphysis pubis. Fluid is infused under gravity and bladder capacity, presence of sensation, and presence of bladder contraction or instability can be identified.

Cystometry also can be performed using a single-channel pressure recording. Single-channel recording produces a measurement of total bladder pressure without accounting for pressure-related phenomenon owing to increases in intra-abdominal pressure. In these cases, the recording catheter may be placed transurethrally or through a temporary suprapubic approach [46]. The catheter has either two or three lumens for infusion and simultaneous bladder pressure measurement (two lumen) or bladder and urethral pressure measurement (three lumen). Because catheter size is shown to produce obstruction to flow, smaller catheters (10F or less) should be used to avoid this [47]. Alternatively, two small catheters may be used, with removal of the infusing catheter before the voiding attempt [48].

Multichannel studies use simultaneous recording of total bladder pressures (p_{ves}) and separate abdominal pressure (p_{abd}) recording via a catheter in the rectum. Alternatively, transvaginal catheters are used to monitor intra-abdominal pressure. Some investigators believe that these recordings are reproducible and accurate [49]; however, catheter dislodgement and inaccurate placement are potential hazards of this technique. The rectal catheter ranges in size from 5F to 10F and may be a balloon type or may be constructed with a feeding catheter with a covering finger cot. The difference between p_{ves} and p_{abd} is termed detrusor or bladder pressure (p_{det}). Subtracted pressure readings assist in the identification of abdominal pressure events and provide true intravesical pressure readings.

In performing the cystometrogram, filling is initiated with patients placed in the supine or sitting position. During the study, patients may be brought to the erect position, although some investigators perform cystometry in this position throughout the study. Filling may be performed by gravity or infusion pump. All transducers are zeroed before the initiation of filling, and a test cough should demonstrate adequate pressure transmission. Pressure line displacement into the urethra and the presence of air in an inadequately flushed system are two common causes of p_{ves} that do not respond to initial zeroing attempts [50]. Patients should be asked to cough several times during the study to check the apparatus and ensure proper pressure transduction.

The normal adult cystometrogram can be divided into four phases (Fig. 4):

Phase 1. The initial pressure rise represents the response of the muscular and viscoelastic properties of the bladder wall to stretch induced by filling. With liquid infusion, the initial filling pressure usually develops gradually to levels between 0 and 8 cm of water in the supine position. With more rapid rates of filling, initially there may be a higher peak, which eventually should level out.

Phase 2. Phase two is known as the tonus limb, and in normal cases, bladder compliance (change in volume/change in pressure) is high and uninterrupted by phasic rises. It is difficult to find stated normal values for compliance, although an arbitrary value of 12.5 mL/cm often is suggested [51].

Phase 3. Phase 3 demonstrates a rise in bladder pressure with further infusion that indicates the exhaustion of the viscoelastic accommodation of the bladder wall.

Phase 4. Phase 4 consists of the initiation of voluntary micturition. It is characterized by increases in detrusor pressure associated with a simultaneous decrease in outlet resistance and subsequent emptying of the bladder. The detrusor contraction should be of adequate magnitude to empty the bladder. Under normal testing circumstances, some individuals may not demonstrate a detrusor contraction, but this does not represent a significant finding unless other pathologic findings are present.

During filling, the following parameters should be noted and recorded: (1) volume at first desire to void, (2) volume at normal desire to void, (3) volume at urgency, (4) maximum cystometric capacity, (5) compliance (change in volume divided by the change in pressure), and (6) presence or absence of involuntary detrusor contractions. During the study, patients should be questioned repeatedly as to whether or not the study reproduces the symptoms under investigation.

Any bladder contraction during filling is considered by many experts to be abnormal. When an involuntary detrusor contraction occurs, note the volume at which it occurs, whether or not it coincides with a sensation of urgency, and whether or not suppression is possible. The sensation of urgency at the time of involuntary activity suggests intact neural pathways in the pelvis and spinal cord.

Fluoroscopic monitoring of bladder filling and contraction further amplifies the results obtained from pressure cystometry. Vesicoureteral reflux can be identified and characterized. The status of the bladder outlet at rest and during contraction is delineated. Incontinence can be related better to the detrusor, the outlet, or a combination of causes. The anatomic appearance of the bladder, including the presence of diverticula or trabeculations and the overall bladder shap, also can be assessed.

Several key issues that can be encountered during the performance of a cystometrogram deserve mention in this discussion: detrusor

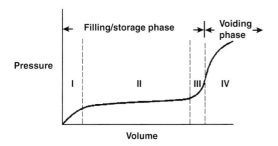

Fig. 4. Schematic of an idealized normal adult cystometrogram. See text for description. (*Adapted from* Dmochowski RR. Cystometry. Urol Clin North Am 1996;23:243–52.)

overactivity (DO), compliance, and leak-point pressures.

Detrusor overactivity

Involuntary detrusor contractions during filling are believed by some experts to be always significant [52]. Originally, the International Continence Society limited the definition of DO to phasic rises in detrusor pressure of greater than 15 cm of water. Clinical experience indicates, however, that involuntary contractions of lesser magnitude often are associated with severe symptoms [53]. Currently, the accepted definition of DO is a phasic rise in detrusor pressure over baseline, no matter what the magnitude, that reproduces the patient's symptoms. The clinical significance of involuntary detrusor activity that does not reproduce symptoms is as yet undefined. Involuntary detrusor contractions are known to occur in healthy, asymptomatic volunteers [54,55] and may be found in up to 68% of patients on ambulatory UDS (Fig. 5) [56].

Several parameters should be noted during an involuntary detrusor contraction. The volume at which DO occurs, the amplitude of the contraction, the duration of the contraction, the associated symptoms, and whether or not leakage occurs or a void is precipitated all are important variables to record. These factors may give information about the severity of the condition or the response to particular therapies; however, there is no objective evidence relating any of these factors to clinical prognosis or response to therapy [41,57].

When unexpected DO is found at a low infused volume that is of questionable clinical significance, the impact of filling rate must be considered, and a slower rate of fill may be attempted [58]. This is not to suggest that unexpected DO is not important or does not have the possibility of being clinically significant; however, it always is important to interpret questionable results in the context of individual patients [52]. When DO is suspected based on patient symptoms but cannot be shown on UDS, provocative measures can be used during a repeat filling phase, such as coughing, Valsalva's maneuver, rapid infusion rates, or a change of position (ie, from seated to standing) [59].

Compliance

Compliance refers to the volume and pressure relationship of bladder filling (change in volume/change in pressure). Three variables affect the compliance capability of the urinary bladder: (1) intravesical pressure, (2) mural tension, and (3) bladder volume. Compliance reflects the bladder's innate ability to expand to capacity with minimal changes in intravesical pressure. This expansile capability is contributed to by the smooth

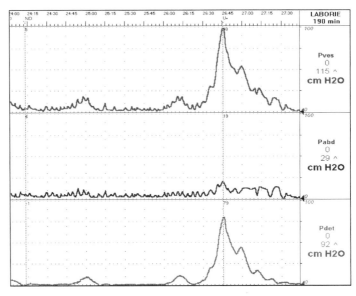

Fig. 5. Urodynamic filling tracing demonstrating high-amplitude involuntary detrusor contraction. (Courtesy of Laborie Medical Technologies, Burlington, VT.)

muscular, collagenous, and elastic components of the bladder submucosa and muscularis [60]. The normally innervated bladder without the presence of coexistent pathologic lesions (eg, infection, fibrosis, or carcinoma) retains this viscoelastic capability during the storage phase of micturition.

Compliance assumes a crucial role in the long-term health of the upper urinary tract. The effects of elevated detrusor pressures on ureteral transport can be significant [61–63]. In myelodysplastic children, a value of 40 cm H_2O is shown to be associated with upper urinary tract deterioration [63]. The intrinsic relationship between compliance and the bladder outlet is demonstrated by successful modulation of infravesical obstruction, which improves compliance [64].

Measured compliance during UDS studies can be affected by infusion rate, the position of the patient, volume of liquid infused, and other factors [41]. Decreased compliance classically is found in several disorders, including myelodysplasia, spinal cord injury, radiation cystitis, post-pelvic surgery, and so forth.

Leak-point pressures

Leak-point pressure testing originated from VUDS studies done over many years in a broad cross-section of patients, including those who have idiopathic incontinence, stress incontinence, and neurogenic conditions. Currently, there are two leak-point pressure tests that measure different aspects of lower urinary tract function [65]. The two tests are not complementary and are used to evaluate conditions in two different patient populations.

Several investigators describe the relationship between p_{det} and urethral outlet resistance at the instant of flow. p_{det} usually is the product of a bladder muscular contraction. With muscular shortening, pressure on the urinary system is developed. Once flow is initiated and continues, p_{det} commonly is related to outlet resistance [66]. A detrusor leak-point pressure (DLPP) is not useful in determining whether or not obstruction exists in non-neurogenic situations nor is it useful in characterizing bladder contractility. The DLPP is simply a measurement of p_{det} when leakage occurs across the urethra, in the absence of an involuntary detrusor contraction or a volitional void [62]. As discussed previously, studies determine that upper tract deterioration is apt to occur when storage occurs at sustained intravesical pressures exceeding 40 cm H_2O. The

concept of DLPP has revolutionized the management of patients who have neurogenic voiding dysfunction, and strict attention to this parameter with the goal of preservation of low intravesical pressures leads to vastly improved outcomes with respect to upper and lower urinary tract function in select patient populations.

Measurement of DLPP is recommended in individuals who have decreased compliance and urinary incontinence. For this test, patients should remain at rest throughout the study and not attempt to void volitionally. The bladder is filled passively until a detrusor contraction is seen, an intravesical pressure of 40 cm H_2O is reached, or leakage occurs around the catheter.

The Valsalva leak-point pressure (VLPP) or abdominal leak-point pressure is an indirect measure of the bladder outlet to resist increases in abdominal pressure [67]. The p_{det} at leakage is representative of the resistance of the urethra to the bladder. VLPP and the DLPP are not the same measurement, as the VLPP is calculated with voluntary abdominal strain. The VLPP generally is used clinically to determine the presence and estimate the severity of sphincteric or stress urinary incontinence. Multichannel studies with a pressure-transducing catheter in the bladder and rectum are useful to estimate the VLPP, as changes in abdominal pressure can be recorded while confirming that detrusor pressure remains constant. The bladder is filled to a predetermined value and patients asked perform a graded Valsalva's maneuver until leakage is seen through the urethra via radiographic confirmation or visual inspection. The pressure at which leakage occurs is recorded as the VLPP.

If leakage is not produced, patients are asked to cough. It is the authors' practice to perform initial VLPP testing at volumes of 150 mL. In patients who cannot hold this volume, it may be necessary to perform testing at smaller volumes. If patients do not demonstrate leakage at 150 mL, the authors typically repeat the evaluation at 250 mL. If patients who complain of stress incontinence still do not leak, testing can be repeated at higher volumes or during refill with the urethral catheter removed. A normal bladder outlet should not leak at any reproducible pressure. In cases where leakage is demonstrated, the numeric value of the VLPP is believed to correlate directly with the degree of bladder outlet function. The higher the VLPP, the better the sphincteric function; conversely, the lower the VLPP, the worse the function. A VLPP of less than 60 to 65 cm H_2O generally is accepted to represent intrinsic sphincteric deficiency [53]. Higher leak-point pressures (>100 cm H_2O) generally are associated with urethral hypermobility, but not always. Other tests or radiographic capabilities are necessary to confirm this association. In cases of patients who have concomitant pelvic organ prolapse, it is recommended that VLPP testing be performed with the prolapse reduced either with a vaginal pack or a pessary to rule out the presence of occult stress incontinence.

VLPP alone does not provide sufficient information for development of a therapeutic plan, but it can help. There still are problems with standardization of technique, specification of variables, sizes of urethral catheters, and the bladder volume at which VLPP is tested.

In summary, cystometry is likened to the reflex hammer of neurourologic testing [12,53,68]. The ability of this tool to reproduce symptoms and to elaborate a diagnosis is dependent on the systematic performance and appropriate modification or cystometry to particular clinical situations.

Pressure-flow analysis

Measurements of urine flow rate and postvoid residual volume can give the clinician valuable information about the voiding phase of micturition, but they do not provide information about the specific nature of existing abnormalities [69]. The main purpose of pressure-flow studies is to identify and in some cases quantify the abnormalities of underlying disorders of voiding. Pressure-flow UDS assesses the interaction of the bladder, bladder outlet, pelvic floor, and urethra during voiding. The use of simultaneous pelvic floor kinesiologic studies (EMG) and simultaneous fluoroscopy are discussed later; they are useful and sometimes indispensable adjuncts for identifying the location of suspected urethral obstruction or confirming neurologic abnormalities [70].

Pressure-flow analysis most often is performed after filling cystometry once maximum bladder capacity is met. Patients are asked to void volitionally while intravesical pressure, intra-abdominal pressure, and flow rate and volume are recorded. For the purposes of proper interpretation, the point at which patients are asked to void should be well documented on the UDS tracing. If patients have an involuntary detrusor contraction during filling that results in a precipitous void, this should not be interpreted as a normal void. Although emptying the bladder as a result of an involuntary

detrusor contraction may resemble a normal void on the UDS tracing, this phenomenon does not necessarily suggest normal emptying and may be representative of significant pathology.

One of the main diagnoses that can be elucidated using pressure-flow studies is bladder outlet obstruction. Urodynamically, obstruction is defined by the relationship between detrusor pressure and flow [52]. A high-pressure void associated with low-urine flow rate implies obstruction (Fig. 6). A low-pressure void in the setting of a low urine flow rate implies impaired detrusor contractility that can be seen with or without associated bladder outlet obstruction. A high-pressure void in the setting of normal flow rates suggests outlet obstruction with a well-compensated detrusor. The normal adult male voids with a detrusor pressure of between 40 and 60 cm of water. A p_{det} higher than this with a Qmax of less than 10 mL per second implies obstruction. Determining normal values for detrusor pressures in adult females is controversial. Females void with much lower pressures than males. In fact, some female patients do not generate a detrusor contraction at all to void. This does not indicate that a detrusor contraction cannot occur, but in some cases that it is not necessary because of low levels of outlet resistance during voiding. Bladder outlet obstruction does exist in females in cases who do and do not have a history of prior surgery. The accepted parameters for diagnosing obstruction in females recently have been proposed to be a detrusor pressure of greater than 20 cm H_2O, accompanied by a flow rate of less than 15 mL per second [71].

As detrusor pressures and flow rates can be highly variable, several nomograms have been developed to assist in making the diagnosis of bladder outlet obstruction [65,72]. These nomograms are sex specific and the most commonly used instruments are validated only for males. The International Continence Society nomogram is the most widely used and accepted in contemporary practice [72]. The pressure-flow diagram is divided into three regions: (1) unobstructed, (2) obstructed, and (3) equivocal. The boundaries between the regions originally were determined from a combination of theoretic analysis and empiric observation. The position of the Qmax point plotted on the diagram determines if the void is unobstructed, obstructed, or equivocal (Fig. 7).

Several sophisticated formulas attempt to calculate a number for outlet resistance. Conversely, the Abrams-Griffiths number is a simple value to

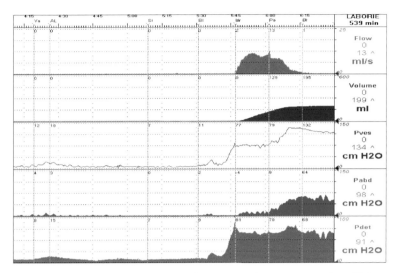

Fig. 6. Pressure-flow urodynamic tracing demonstrating high-pressure detrusor contraction with low to moderate flow caused by bladder outlet obstruction in a male. (Courtesy of Laborie Medical Technologies, Burlington, VT.)

calculate and can be used to determine rapidly if a given pressure-flow study represents obstruction [73]. The number is calculated as follows:

Abrams-Griffiths number

$= p_{det}Qmax - 2 Qmax$

$p_{det}Qmax$

$=$ detrusor pressure at maximum flow

If the Abrams-Griffiths number is greater than 40, it is likely that patients are obstructed; if less than 15, patients likely are unobstructed; if between 15 and 40, the results are considered equivocal and diagnosis may be based on clinical presentation and other testing modalities.

The strength of the detrusor contraction also can be determined via pressure-flow testing. As discussed previously, voids with low p_{det} and low Q_{max} correspond to a weak detrusor contraction. p_{det} and flow rate should be considered when diagnosing detrusor hypocontractility. A low p_{det} with an adequate or high flow rate actually may correspond to a normal or strong detrusor contraction. Schaefer suggests a nomogram to characterize strength of detrusor contraction. Straight lines divide the pressure-flow diagram into regions labeled very weak, weak, normal, and strong [65]. This simple and approximate grading into four classes is easy to carry out in combination with a graphic method, such as the Abrams-Griffiths or the International Continence Society nomogram (Fig. 8).

Pressure-flow studies of voiding offer the only unambiguous way of assessing bladder outlet obstruction and detrusor contractility. The methods of analysis yield results that broadly are consistent. The most important aspect of pressure-flow studies is the quality of the information obtained. This implies that good technique and judgment be used while performing a study and that a study adequately represents normal and abnormal aspects of a typical voiding event.

Electromyography

EMG is a portion of UDS studies that enables urologists to evaluate the striated sphincter and pelvic floor during bladder filling and emptying. Kinesiologic EMG enables examiners to determine if the striated sphincteric complex appropriately increases its activity in a gradual fashion during bladder filling and if there is appropriate relaxation before and during the voiding phase [48,74]. EMG can be performed either with needle electrodes or surface or patch electrodes. Needle electrodes provide more accurate placement and recording; however, they are significantly more invasive, and patch electrodes in most cases provide the necessary information.

Normally, as the bladder fills with urine, there is a gradual and sustained increase in EMG activity, a phenomenon known as the guarding reflex. EMG activity should reach its height just before voiding. The lack of a guarding reflex may indicate neural pathology. Voluntary voiding

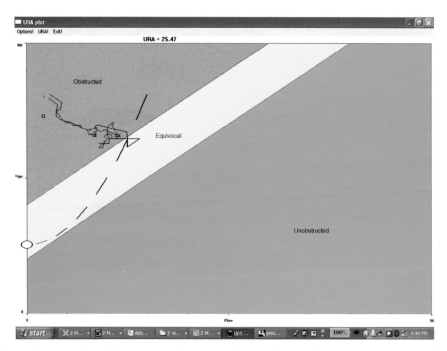

Fig. 7. Example of an ICS nomogram. (Courtesy of Laborie Medical Technologies, Burlington, VT.)

normally is preceded by EMG silence, representing relaxation of the striated sphincter and pelvic floor.

Several factors that can result in increased EMG activity during filling include abdominal straining, coughing, crede, Valsalva's maneuver, and involuntary detrusor contractions. Increased EMG activity during voiding should be interpreted carefully (Fig. 9). It can be the result of patients attempting to suppress voiding, increased pelvic floor tone during voiding as seen in dysfunctional voiding patients, or a true neurologic lesion resulting in detrusor-sphincter dyssynergia [52], which refers to the obstruction of outflow of urine during a bladder contraction caused by involuntary contraction of the striated sphincter. True detrusor-sphincter dyssynergia is exceedingly rare in a neurologically normal individual, and such a diagnosis deserves exhaustive study before it is confirmed [75,76].

Videourodynamics

The previous discussion detailed UDS as the primary method of studying the physiology of the lower urinary tract. When these studies are combined with an imaging technique, such as VUDS, the anatomy and physiology of the lower urinary tract can be evaluated simultaneously.

The ability of the clinician to visualize the anatomy of the urinary tract at specific moments during physiologic micturition results in the most comprehensive and complete examination used to study the anatomy and physiology of voiding and voiding dysfunction [17].

During the past 40 years, VUDS has become far more than a research tool. With technical advances in computer software and hardware and imaging equipment combined with decreased costs and increased portability, VUDS has become more accessible and is found in many office settings.

The factor that sets VUDS apart from standard UDS is the imaging component. VUDS is performed most commonly with fluoroscopy; however, some investigators claim real-time ultrasonography to be of equivalent value [77–79]. At the authors' institution, digitally acquired fluoroscopy is used to monitor the filling and storage and the voiding phases of the micturition cycle intermittently, ultimately comprising a complete voiding cystourethrogram at the close of the test. Some centers use a fixed fluoroscopy unit and some use C-arm fluoroscopy. With either set-up, the amount of radiation used in every case should be limited. In most cases, 1 minute or less of fluoroscopy time is necessary to complete

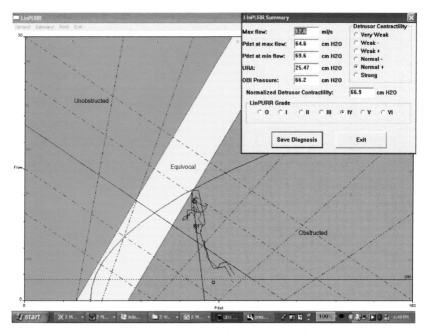

Fig. 8. Example of a Schaefer nomogram. (Courtesy of Laborie Medical Technologies, Burlington, VT.)

a study [80]. Despite multiple variables in VUDS techniques, when the standardized portions of the test are adhered to, the results are highly reproducible.

VUDS should be performed as described previously for UDS studies. On initial presentation, a scout film should be obtained before the positioning of patients and placement of the pressure transducing catheters. Studies may be performed either in the standing or seated position, depending on the presenting abnormalities and on the capabilities of the laboratory. Patients who have significant neurologic disabilities may need to be evaluated in a recumbent oblique position. Urethral and rectal catheters then are placed and their positions confirmed with a repeat KUB. After pressure equalization and zeroing of the transducers, a noniodinated radio-opaque solution is used to fill the bladder at previously recommended fill rates. VUDS studies should progress in the same manner as routine pressure-flow UDS studies. During bladder filling, provocative maneuvers are performed, such as Valsalva's maneuver and cough, and are repeated in an attempt to recreate the symptoms. Valsalva's maneuver and (when applicable) DLLPs are assessed and recorded. Leakage of urine as a result of involuntary detrusor activity, impaired compliance, and stress maneuvers are recorded. During

the investigation, rest and strain images are captured periodically and with each provocative maneuver to assess the competence and mobility of the bladder base, bladder neck, and urethra. Additional images are obtained as needed to evaluate vesicoureteral reflux, bladder or urethral calculi, fistulae, intravesical or intraurethral filling defects, and bladder or urethral diverticula (Figs. 10 and 11). When bladder capacity is reached, patients are asked to void volitionally, and they void into the uroflowmeter under fluoroscopic guidance. Multiple images are exposed during voiding to evaluate the bladder neck and urethra, ensuring adequate opening and ruling out anatomic obstruction (Figs. 12 and 13). Additional images are obtained to document the presence or absence of vesicoureteral reflux. At the conclusion of the voiding phase, a postvoid image is obtained to again assess vesicoureteral reflux, bladder or urethral diverticula, and so forth [17].

Urodynamic coding

In general, coding for UDS in the office setting includes a cluster of descriptors that includes complex uroflowmetry, cystometrogram, and voiding pressure studies. These codes should be listed separately as discrete and granular (separately identifiable) procedures when performed in

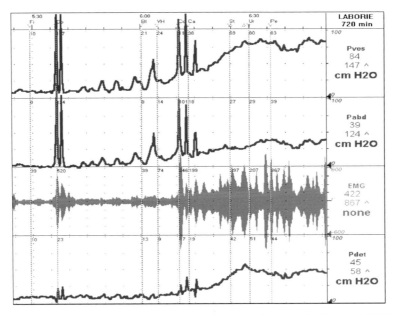

Fig. 9. Urodynamic tracing suspicious for detrusor-sphincter dyssynergia. Note the increased EMG activity during voiding. (Courtesy of Laborie Medical Technologies, Burlington, VT.)

the office setting. In general, professional fees rendered for these codes are somewhat lower in the office setting; however, this professional fee reduction is offset by technical fees that are included when the procedures are performed in an established institutional setting (such as a hospital). These codes currently are not included within the ambulatory surgery setting and, therefore, are limited to either institutional or outpatient office-type venues.

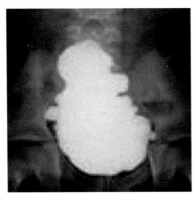

Fig. 10. Fluoroscopic image obtained during filling phase that demonstrates a severely trabeculated neurogenic appearing bladder.

Although the UDS interventions discussed previously usually are performed in sequence and at the same time, they are subject to reductions in reimbursement based on multiple procedures at same setting rules. This reduction is defined clearly for Medicare beneficiaries and less so for third-party payers. Interested physicians are urged to consult with individual payers regarding discrete elements of the complex UDS evaluation for issues regarding reimbursement and specific codes and payment for such.

Codes of interest for the office setting include: 51726 (complex cystometrogram), 51741 (complex uroflowmetry); 51772 (urethral pressure profile studies); 51784 (EMG); 51785 (needle EMG); and 51795/51797 (voiding pressure studies). Recent approval of the 51798 code (postvoid residual) also has occurred.

Each of these codes is used within a specific scenario as follows [81,82].

51726 (Complex cystometrogram)

This is the study that most physicians associate with the in-office UDS evaluation. It involves simultaneous infusion of either saline or contrast while monitoring pressure. This usually, although not necessarily, is done in a setting of simultaneous rectal pressure evaluation. The purpose of

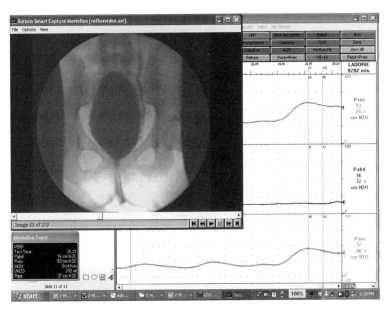

Fig. 11. Fluoroscopic image demonstrating vesicoureteral reflux. (Courtesy of Laborie Medical Technologies, Burlington, VT.)

the complex cystometrogram is to measure bladder filling pressures, sensation, and compliance during the storage cycle of bladder function. Usually at least one pressure channel is monitored, although three and five channel studies are performed most commonly. Oftentimes, this study is amplified with fluoroscopy in a video cystometrogram –type analysis.

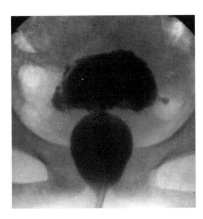

Fig. 12. Fluoroscopic image obtained during VUDS study of a 36- year-old paraplegic female. The image demonstrates a small capacity trabeculated bladder, with distention of the proximal urethra during an involuntary detrusor contraction consistent with striated sphincter dyssynergia.

51741 (Complex uroflowmetry)

This is a standard uroflow study using calibrated electronic equipment and commonly is performed in many specialists' offices for evaluation of peak and mean uroflow rates. The study often is done simultaneously with code 51798 as a measure of distinct bladder emptying function.

51772 (Urethral pressure profile studies)

These studies classically are performed using a urethral catheter across the urethral sphincter mechanism and evaluating functional urethral length and maximum urethral closure pressures,

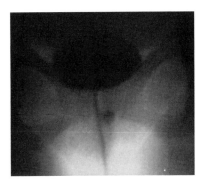

Fig. 13. Fluoroscopic image obtained during voiding demonstrating a urethral diverticulum.

at rest and under stress conditions with the bladder full. Recent changes in the understanding of urethral function have led to the use of VLPP as another analysis of urethral function. VLPP is a measure of urethral function and often is coded using this technique, as it also represents a measure of intrinsic urethral function. The development of new retrograde urethral functional measures has added further to the assessment of urethral function. The urethral retroresistance pressure is described as a technique that measures urethral closure using retrograde pressure measurement [1,2]. Although novel, further standardization and validation of this technique are necessary.

51784/51785 (EMG studies of anal or urethral sphincter, other than needle, any technique [51784]; of anal or urethral sphincter, any technique [51785])

Most centers use skin patch electrodes for EMG monitoring. The use of electrodes often is complicated by problems with moisture on the skin or poor adherence, making interpretation difficult. EMG, however, is crucial in those circumstances where analysis for voiding dysfunction possibly associated with a dyssynergic (true neurologic component) or pseudodyssynergic voiding pattern (non-neurologic) is necessary. Needle EMG is considered the gold standard comparator study; however, this method represents substantive patient discomfort and can be approximated with patch electrode studies in most circumstances.

51795/51797 (Voiding pressure studies, any technique [51795] and intra-abdominal voiding pressure using either rectal gastric or intraperitoneal measurements [51797])

Voiding pressure studies are a crucial aspect of the complete UDS evaluation and should be considered as an included component in all studies when urinary symptoms, especially outlet urinary symptoms, are associated with the presenting vignette. Voiding studies can be performed using either a measurement of bladder pressure during the voiding event (as assessed with a urethral catheter) or with simultaneous intrarectal or vaginal pressures so that subtracted pressures may be obtained. These measures represent the most accurate means of determining true voiding pressure and allow an assessment of voiding dynamics, not only of outlet obstruction but also as an estimation of detrusor contraction.

Summary

UDS studies represent a vital and intrinsic component of outpatient urologic assessment. Improvements in testing methodology and equipment have made these studies attractive to many general urologists, gynecologists, and other specialists. Use of these methods must be carefully monitored, however, as they bear significant burden to health care expenditure and also impart some level of patient discomfiture and inconvenience. Therefore, a specific group of circumstances should be used as indications for the performance of UDS. Nonetheless, UDS serve a vital role as an objectification of subjective symptoms and, in the authors' practice, is performed before any procedure with permanent connotations or in circumstances of diagnostic quandary.

References

[1] Rose DK. Determination of bladder pressures with the cystometer. JAMA 1927;88:151–3.
[2] Drake WM. The uroflowmeter: an aid to the study of the lower urinary tract. J Urol 1948;59:650.
[3] von Garrelts B. Analysis of micturition. A new method of recording the voiding of the bladder. Acta Chir Scand 1956;112:326–7.
[4] Franksson C, Peterson I. Electromyographic investigation of disturbances of the striated muscle of the urethral sphincter. Br J Urol 1955;27:154–7.
[5] Miller ER. X-ray movies. Radiology 1954;63:571 [editorial].
[6] Miller ER. Techniques for the simultaneous display of X-ray and physiologic data. In: Boyarsky S, editor. The neurogenic bladder. Baltimore: Williams & Wilkins; 1967. p. 79.
[7] Turner-Warwick R, Whiteside CG. Clinical urodynamics. Urol Clin North Am 1979;6:1–18.
[8] Rovner ES, Wein AJ. Practical urodynamics: part I. AUA Update Series. Vol. XXI, Lesson 19; 2002.
[9] Nitti VW, editor. Practical urodynamics. Phildelphia: W.B. Saunders; 1998.
[10] Blaivas J, Chancellor M. Atlas of urodynamics. Baltimore: Williams & Wilkins; 1996.
[11] Mundy AR, Stephenson TP, Wein AJ, editors. Urodynamics: principles, practice and application. New York: Churchill Livingstone; 1984.
[12] Blaivas JG. Management of bladder dysfunction in multiple sclerosis. Neurology 1980;30(7 pt 2):12–8.
[13] Seaman EK, Jacobs BZ, Blaivas JG, et al. Persistence or recurrence of symptoms after transurethral resection of the prostate: a urodynamic assessment. J Urol 1994;152:935–7.
[14] Katz GP, Blaivas JG. A diagnostic dilemma: when urodynamic findings differ from the clinical impression. J Urol 1983;129:1170–4.

[15] James M, Jackson S, Shepard A, et al. Pure stress leakage symptomatology: is it safe to discount detrusor instability? Br J Obstet Gynecol 1999;106:1255–8.

[16] Abrams P. New word for old: lower urinary tract symptoms for "prostatism." BMJ 1994;308:929–30.

[17] Rovner ES, Banner MP, Ramchandani P, et al. Clinical videourodynamics. AUA Update Series Vol. XXII, Lesson 35; 2003.

[18] Klinger HC, Maderbacher S, Djavan B, et al. Morbidity of the evaluation of the lower urinary tract with trans-urethral multi-channel pressure-flow studies. J Urol 1998;159:191–4.

[19] Talbot GH, Doorley M, Banner MP. Urosepsis associated with urodynamic studies. Am J Infect Control 1984;12:266–70.

[20] McConnell JD. Why pressure-flow studies should be optional and not mandatory studies for evaluating men with benign prostatic hyperplasia. Urology 1994;44:156–8.

[21] Wein AJ. Neuromuscular dysfunction of the lower urinary tract and its treatment. In: Walsh PC, Retik A, Vaughn E, Wein AJ, editors. Campbells urology. 7th edition. Philadelphia: W.B. Saunders; 1998. p. 953–1006.

[22] Abrams P, Torrens M. Urine flow studies. Urol Clin North Am 1979;6:71–8.

[23] Christmas TJ, Chapple CR, Rickards D, et al. Contemporary flowmeters: an assessment of their accuracy and reliability. Br J Urol 1989;63:460–71.

[24] Nielson JB, Norgaard JP, Sorenson SS, et al. Continuous overnight monitoring of bladder activity in vesico-ureteral reflux patients: II. Bladder activity types. Neurourol Urodynam 1984;3:7–10.

[25] Van De Beek C, Stoevelaar HJ, McDonnel J, et al. Interpretation of uroflowmetry curves by urologists. J Urol 1997;157:164–8.

[26] Golomb J, Lindner A, Seigel Y, et al. Variability and circadian changes in home uroflometry in patient with benign prostatic hyperplasia compared to normal controls. J Urol 1992;147:1044.

[27] Feneley MR, Dunsmuir WD, Pearce J, et al. Reproducibility of uroflow measurement: Experience during a double blind, placebo controlled study of doxasosin in benign prostatic hyperplasia. Urology 1996;47:658–63.

[28] Jorgensen JB, Jensen KB. Uroflowmetry. Urol Clin North Am 1996;23:237–42.

[29] Drach GW, Layton TN, Binard WJ. Male peak urinary flow rate: relationships to volume and age. J Urol 1979;122:215–8.

[30] Abrams P. Prostatism and prostatectomy: the value of urine flow rate measurement in the pre-operative assessment for operation. J Urol 1977;117:70–4.

[31] Anderson JT, Jacobson O, Worm-Peterson J, et al. Bladder function in healthy elderly males. Scan J Urol Nephrol 1978;12:123–5.

[32] Anikwe RM. Urinary flow rate in benign prostatic hypertrophy. Int Surg 1976;61:109–13.

[33] Anikwe RM. Urodynamics in benign prostatic hypertrophy. Br J Urol 1978;50:20–4.

[34] Ball AJ, Smith PJ. Urodynamic factors in relation to outcome of prostatectomy. Urology 1986;28:256–8.

[35] Bottacini MR, Gleason DM. Urodynamic norms in women: normal versus stress incontinence. J Urol 1980;124:659–61.

[36] Drach GW, Ignatoff J, Layton T. Peak urinary flow rate: observations in female subjects and comparison to male subjects. J Urol 1979;122:215–9.

[37] Frimodt-Moller C, Hald T. Clinical urodynamics. Methods and results. Scand J Urol Nephrol 1972;6(Suppl 15):144–54.

[38] Gleason DM, Bottacini MR. Urodynamic norms in female voiding: the flow modulating zone and voiding dysfunction. J Urol 1982;127:495–8.

[39] Susset JG. Relationship between clinical urodynamics and pathologic findings in prostatic obstruction. In: Hinman F Jr, editor. Benign prostatic hyperplasia. New York: Springer Verlag; 1983. p. 613.

[40] Tanagho EA, Stoller ML. Urodynamics: uroflowmetry and female voiding patterns. In: Oestergard DR, Bent AE, editors. Urogynecology and urodynamics. Baltimore: Williams & Wilkins; 1991. p. 346.

[41] Homma Y, Batista JE, Bauer SB, et al. Urodynamics. In: Abrams P, Khoury S, Wein AJ, editors. Incontinence. Plymouth, United Kingdom: Health Publication; 1999. p. 353–400.

[42] Aslund K, Rentzhogh L, Sandstromb G. Effects of ice cold saline and acid solution in urodynamics. In: Proceedings of the 18th Annual Meeting of the International Continence Society. Oslo, Norway. New York (NY): Alan R. Liss. 1988. p. 1–4.

[43] Sethia KK, Smith JC. The effect of pH and lignocaine on detrusor instability. Br J Urol 1987;60:516–8.

[44] Bates P, Bradley WE, Glen E, et al. First report on the standardization of terminology of lower urinary tract function. Br J Urol 1976;48:39–41.

[45] Dmochowski RR. Cystometry. Urol Clin North Am 1996;23:243–52.

[46] Rollema HJ, van Mastright R, Ambergen AW, et al. Detrusor instability in benign prostatic hypertrophy (BPH); low incidence by suprapubic filling cystometry. Neurourol Urodynam 1990;9:422–8.

[47] Tessier J, Schick E. Does urethral instrumentation affect uroflowmetry measurements? Br J Urol 1990;65:261–6.

[48] Wein AJ, English WE, Whitmore KE. Office urodynamics. Urol Clin North Am 1988;15:609–16.

[49] James ED, Niblett PG, MacNaughton JA, et al. The vagina as alternative to the rectum in measuring abdominal pressure during urodynamic investigations. Br J Urol 1987;60:212–6.

[50] Stephenson TP. The interpretation of conventional urodynamics. In: Mundy AR, Stephenson TP,

Wein AJ, editors. Urodynamics: principles, practice, and application. Edinburgh (Scotland): Churchill Livingstone; 1994. p. 113.

[51] Toppercer A, Tetreault JP. Compliance of the bladder: an attempt to establish normal values. Urology 1979;14:204.

[52] Rovner ES, Wein AJ. Practical urodynamics: part II. AUA Update Series. Vol. XXI, Lesson 20; 2002.

[53] Blaivas JG. Techniques of evaluation. In: Yalla SV, McGuire EJ, Elbadawi A, et al, editors. Neurology and urodynamics, principles and practice. New York: Macmillan Publishing; 1988. p. 155–98.

[54] van Waalwijk van Doorn ES, Meier AH, Ambergen AW, et al. Ambulatory urodynamics: extramural testing of the lower and upper urinary tract by Holter monitoring of cystometrogram, uroflometry, and renal pelvic pressure. Urol Clin North Am 1996;23: 345–71.

[55] Wyndaele JJ. Normality in urodynamics studies in healthy adults. J Urol 1999;161:899–902.

[56] Heslington K, Hilton P. Ambulatory monitoring and conventional cystometry in asymptomatic female volunteers. Br J Obstet Gynecol 1996;103: 434–41.

[57] Wagg A, Bayliss M, Ingham NJ, et al. Urodynamic variables cannot be used to classify the severity of detrusor instability. Br J Urol 1998;82: 499–502.

[58] Nitti VW. Cystometry and abdominal pressure monitoring. In: Nitti VW, editor. Practical urodynamics. Philadelphia: W.B. Saunders; 1998. p. 38–51.

[59] Choe JM, Gallo MK, Staskin DR. A provocative maneuver to elicit cystometric instability: Measuring instability at maximum infusion. J Urol 1999;161: 1541–4.

[60] Churchill BM, Gilmour RF, Williot P. Urodynamics. Pediatr Clin North Am 1987;34:1133–5.

[61] McGuire EM. Bladder compliance [editorial]. J Urol 1994;151:965.

[62] Mcguire EM, Woodside JR, Borden TA. Prognostic value of urodynamic testing in myelodysplastic children. J Urol 1981;126:205–7.

[63] McGuire EM, Woodside JR, Borden TA. Upper urinary tract deterioration in patients with myelodysplasia and detrusor hypertonia: a follow-up study. J Urol 1983;129:183–7.

[64] Bloom DA, Knechtel JM, McGuire EM. Urethral dilation improves bladder compliance in children with myelomenigocele and high leak-point pressures. J Urol 1993;144:430–4.

[65] Schaefer W. Basic principles and clinical application of advanced analysis of bladder voiding function. Urol Clin North Am 1990;17:553.

[66] Griffiths DJ, VanMastrier R. The routine assessment of detrusor contraction strength. Neurourol Urodn 1985;4:77–80.

[67] McGuire E, Cespedes D, O'Connell HE. Leak point pressures. Urol Clin North Am 1996;23:253–62.

[68] Blaivas JG. Multichannel urodynamic studies in men with benign prostatic hyperplasia: Indications and interpretation. Urol Clin North Am 1990;17: 543–55.

[69] Griffiths DJ, Scholtmeijer RJ. Place of the free flow curve in the urodynamic evaluation of children. Br J Urol 1984;56:474–8.

[70] Griffiths DJ. Pressure-flow studies of micturition. Urol Clin North Am 1996;23:279–97.

[71] Chassagne S, Bernier PA, Haab F, et al. Proposed cutoff values to define bladder outlet obstruction in women. Urology 1998;51:408–11.

[72] Abrams P, Griffiths PJ. The assessment of prostatic obstruction from urodynamic measurements and from residual urine. Br J Urol 1979;51:129.

[73] Lim CS, Abrams P. The Abrams-Griffith nomogram. World J Urol 1995;13:34–9.

[74] Wein AJ, Barrett DM. Voiding function and dysfunction: a logical and practical approach. Chicago: Year Book Medical Publishers; 1988.

[75] Blaivas JG, Sinha HP, Zayed AA, et al. Detrusor-external sphincter dyssynergia: a detailed electromyographic study. J Urol 1982;127:949.

[76] Blaivas JG, Sinha HP, Zayed AA, et al. Detrusor-external sphincter dyssynergia. J Urol 1981;125: 542–4.

[77] Koebl H, Bernaschek G. A new method for sonographic urethrocystography and simultaneous pressure-flow measurements. Obstet Gynecol 1989; 74:417–22.

[78] Shabsigh R, Fishman IJ, Kreb M. Combined transrectal ultrasonography and urodynamics in the evaluation of detrusor-sphincter dyssynergia. Br J Urol 1988;62:326–30.

[79] Bidair M, Tiechman JM, Brodak PP, et al. Transrectal ultrasound urodynamics. Urology 1993;42:640–4.

[80] Webster GD, Kreder KJ. The neurourologic evaluation. In: Walsh PC, Retik A, Vaughan ED, Wein A, editors. Campbells urology. 7th edition. Philadelphia: W.B. Saunders; 1998. p. 927–52.

[81] Slack M, Tracey M, Hunsicker K, et al. Urethral retro-resistance pressure: a new clinical measure of urethral function. Neurourol Urodynam 2004;23: 656–61.

[82] Slack M, Culligan P, Tracey M, et al. Relationship of urethral retro-resistance pressure to urodynamic measurements of incontinence severity. Neurourol Urodynam 2004;23:109–14.

ELSEVIER
SAUNDERS

Urol Clin N Am 32 (2005) 371–377

UROLOGIC
CLINICS
of North America

Index

Note: Page numbers of article titles are in **boldface** type.

A

Ablation, tissue, office-based procedures for, in benign prostatic hyperplasia, **327–335**

Accountants, role of in urologic practice, **263–269**
    capital improvements, 265
    choice of business entity, 263–264
        C corporation, 263
        limited liability company or partnership, 263
        partnership, 263
        S corporation, 264
        sole proprietor, 263
    depreciation methods, 265–266
    other tax considerations, 268–269
        alternative minimum tax planning, 269
        in divorce, 268–269
    practice compensation models, 264–265
        base salary plus incentive, 264–265
        compensation divided equally, 264
        part equal, part productivity, 264
        productivity, 264
    tax laws and tax strategies, 266–268
        capital gains rates, 267
        charitable deductions of vehicles, 266–267
        health savings accounts, 267–268
        marriage relief penalty, 267

Accrual basis accounting, 296

Acute scrotum, office-based ultrasound of, 348

Age Discrimination in Employment Act, 258

Alternative minimum tax planning, 269

American Academy of Professional Coders, 289

American Health Information Management System, 289

American Urological Association, services for coding and reimbursement, 287–288

Americans with Disabilities Act, 256–257

B

Balloon-based thermotherapy, urethral fluid, for benign prostatic hyperplasia, 331–332

Benefits, retirement plans, for physicians and employees, 269, **309–317**

Benign prostatic hyperplasia, office-based procedures for, **327–335**
    interstitial laser coagulation, 331
    intraprostatic injection for, 330–331
    transrectal ultrasound (TRUS), 332–333
    transurethral microwave thermotherapy (TUMT), 327–328
    transurethral needle ablation (TUNA), 328–330
    urethral fluid balloon-based thermotherapy, 331–332

Bladder, office-based ultrasound of, 342–344
    masses, 343–344
    residual urine, 344
    urodynamics, 344
    office-based urodynamic studies of, **353–370**

Budgeting, for urologic practices, **294–297**
    budget components, 295–296
        capital, 296
        expense, 295
        operating, 295–296
        revenue, 295
    cash *versus* accrual basis accounting, 296
    reasons for, 294–295
    using the budget and financial statements, 296–297

Budgets, components of, 295–296
    capital, 296
    expense, 295
    operating, 295–296
    revenue, 295

Business entity, choice of, for urologic practice, 263–264

0094-0143/05/$ - see front matter © 2005 Elsevier Inc. All rights reserved.
doi:10.1016/S0094-0143(05)00071-6

Changing Your Address?

Make sure your subscription changes too! When you notify us of your new address, you can help make our job easier by including an exact copy of your Clinics label number with your old address (see illustration below.) This number identifies you to our computer system and will speed the processing of your address change. Please be sure this label number accompanies your old address and your corrected address—you can send an old Clinics label with your number on it or just copy it exactly and send it to the address listed below.

We appreciate your help in our attempt to give you continuous coverage. Thank you.

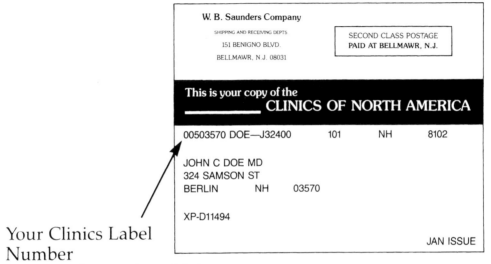

W. B. Saunders Company

SHIPPING AND RECEIVING DEPTS

151 BENIGNO BLVD.

BELLMAWR, N.J. 08031

SECOND CLASS POSTAGE
PAID AT BELLMAWR, N.J.

This is your copy of the
CLINICS OF NORTH AMERICA

00503570 DOE—J32400   101   NH   8102

JOHN C DOE MD
324 SAMSON ST
BERLIN   NH   03570

XP-D11494

JAN ISSUE

Your Clinics Label Number
Copy it exactly or send your label
along with your address to:
W.B. Saunders Company, Customer Service
Orlando, FL 32887-4800
Call Toll Free 1-800-654-2452

Please allow four to six weeks for delivery of new subscriptions and for processing address changes.